Nicola Russo
Sabino Iliceto
Fabio Bellotto

Preventive Cardiology and Rehabilitation

Impressum / Stampa

Bibliografische Information der Deutschen Nationalbibliothek: Die Deutsche Nationalbibliothek verzeichnet diese Publikation in der Deutschen Nationalbibliografie; detaillierte bibliografische Daten sind im Internet über http://dnb.d-nb.de abrufbar.
Alle in diesem Buch genannten Marken und Produktnamen unterliegen warenzeichen-, marken- oder patentrechtlichem Schutz bzw. sind Warenzeichen oder eingetragene Warenzeichen der jeweiligen Inhaber. Die Wiedergabe von Marken, Produktnamen, Gebrauchsnamen, Handelsnamen, Warenbezeichnungen u.s.w. in diesem Werk berechtigt auch ohne besondere Kennzeichnung nicht zu der Annahme, dass solche Namen im Sinne der Warenzeichen- und Markenschutzgesetzgebung als frei zu betrachten wären und daher von jedermann benutzt werden dürften.

Informazione bibliografica pubblicata da Deutsche Nationalbibliothek (Biblioteca Nazionale Tedesca): la Deutsche Nationalbibliothek novera questa pubblicazione su Deutsche Nationalbibliografie. Dati bibliografici più dettagliati sono disponibili in internet al sito web http://dnb.d-nb.de.
Tutti i nomi di marchi e di prodotti riportati in questo libro sono protetti dalla normativa sul diritto d'Autore e dalla normativa a tutela dei marchi. Questi appartengono esclusivamente ai legittimi proprietari. L'uso di nomi di marchi, di nomi di prodotti, di nomi famosi, di nomi commerciali, di descrizioni dei prodotti, ecc. anche se trovati senza un particolare contrassegno in queste pubblicazioni, sono considerati violazione del diritto d'autore e pertanto non possono essere utilizzati da chiunque.

Coverbild / Immagine di copertina: www.ingimage.com

Verlag / Editore:
Edizioni Accademiche Italiane
ist ein Imprint der / è un marchio di
OmniScriptum GmbH & Co. KG
Heinrich-Böcking-Str. 6-8, 66121 Saarbrücken, Deutschland / Germania
Email / Posta Elettronica: info@edizioni-ai.com

Herstellung: siehe letzte Seite /
Pubblicato: vedi ultima pagina
ISBN: 978-3-639-77686-7

Zugl. / Approved by: Padova, Università degli Studi di Padova, 2014

Nicola Russo
Sabino Iliceto
Fabio Bellotto

Preventive Cardiology and Rehabilitation

New insights in an emerging field

Edizioni Accademiche Italiane

Index

Preventive Cardiology and Rehabilitation

Background: Despite the favourable effects of new therapeutic approaches during the acute phase of cardiac diseases and consequent favourable short-term outcomes, post-acute management and long term prognosis still remain unsatisfactory. Cardiac rehabilitation (CR) is a multidisciplinary treatment with established beneficial effects for the vast majority of cardiac patients and universally considered an important aspect of secondary prevention. Although it has been shown to reduce both morbidity and mortality and it is a class I recommendation in the guidelines, its use remains still rather limited in Europe and in the rest of the world.

Aim: The aim of this PhD research was to examine some aspects still little known, or unknown at all, in this field. In particular, the research aimed to evaluate safety and efficacy of a structured, exercise-based, CR in specific cohorts of patients: after transcatheter aortic valve implantation (TAVI), after left ventricular assist device (LVAD) implantation, and early after an acute myocardial infarction (AMI) in high risk subjects.

Methods: All patients (78 TAVI, mean age 82.1±3.6 years, 42 LVAD, 63.4 ± 7.4 years, and 376 AMI, 64.4±12.3 years) were referred to the Institute Codivilla-Putti (in Cortina d'Ampezzo, BL, Italy) for a two week, in-hospital, CR training and comprehensive risk factors interventions early after the acute event (within two weeks TAVI and AMI, within two months after LVAD implantation).

TAVI patients were compared with 80 consecutive peer patients who were admitted for CR in the same period after surgical aortic valve replacement (sAVR) and LVAD patients compared with 47 coeval chronic heart failure (CHF) patients who were admitted for CR in the same period after an acute heart failure event. In LVAD cohort, cardiac autonomic function was evaluated by means of heart rate variability.

AMI patients were divided into 2 groups according to a 40% left ventricular ejection fraction (LVEF) cut-off at enrolment, in order to evaluate the influence of a reduced LVEF on the rehabilitative process; furthermore, in 326 patients a glucometabolic characterization was obtained by means of a standard oral glucose tolerance test (OGTT) in patients without known diabetes.

In all patients the training protocol consisted of a low-medium intensity exercise protocol developed in three sets of exercises, 6 days per week: 30 min of respiratory workout, followed by an aerobic session on a cyclette (or on an arm ergometer in those patients who were not able to cycle) in the morning and, in the afternoon, 30 min of callisthenic exercises. Each session was supervised by a physician and a physiotherapist and all patients were ECG monitored by a telemetry system.

Functional capacity was assessed by a six min walking test (6MWT) on admission, and a second test at discharge; when possible, a cardiopulmonary exercise test (CPET) was also performed. The Barthel Index (BI) was used as an autonomy index in TAVI and LVAD cohorts. In AMI patients rate of death, hospitalizations, smoke cessation, physical activity and adherence to pharmacological treatment were recorded at follow up (up to 5 years, median 2 years).

Results: Despite the high risk profile of the population, the drop out rate was quite low (1.3% of TAVI, 1.1% of AMI and 11.9% of LVAD patients had to be transferred due to non fatal complications). All the subjects who completed the program had enhanced independence, mobility and functional capacity (mean BI increment was 9.9 ± 12.6, $p < 0.01$ and 11.9 ± 10.5, $p < 0.01$, in TAVI and LVAD patients respectively; mean 6MWT gain was 60.4 ± 46.4 mt, $p < 0.01$, 83.2 ± 36.0 mt, $p < 0.05$, 70.7 ± 55.7 mt, $p < 0.01$, in TAVI, LVAD and AMI patients, respectively).

Analysing the specific cohorts, a smaller proportion of TAVI patients, compared with sAVR, was able to complete at least a 6MWT (82% vs 92%)

4

or a CPET (61% vs 95%) but, in those who did, the distance walked at 6MWT at discharge did not significantly differ between the groups (272.7±108 vs. 294.2±101 mt, p=0.42), neither did the exercise capacity assessed by CPET (peak-VO_2 12.5±3.6 vs. 13.9±2.7 ml/kg/min, p=0.16).

At the end of the program, physical performance in LVAD patients was still generally poor, but not dissimilar from that found in CHF patients (peak-VO_2 reached at CPET was 12.5±3.0 vs. 13.6±2.9 ml/kg/min, p=0.20).

Evaluating AMI patients, subjects with LVEF<40% achieved significantly lower peak-VO_2 at CPET than the controls (15.2±3.9 vs. 18.2±5.2 ml/kg/min, p<0.01). After OGTT administration, a high prevalence of abnormal glucose metabolism was found (54%). As expected, exercise capacity was poorer in diabetic and pre-diabetic patients when compared with normoglicemic (peak-VO_2 at CPET 15.3±4.1 vs 17.9±4.8 vs 19.4±5.5 ml/kg/min, p<0.01). At follow up 73% of the subjects reported to exercise regularly, 77% of the smokers definitively quitted and a high adherence to the therapy was registered. Cardiac and all cause mortality resulted 5.0% and 8.0 % at 1 year and 8.0 % and 13.0 % at 5 years, respectively and resulted higher in older people and in those with lower LVEF.

Conclusions: Patients who underwent TAVI and LVAD implantation are characterized by a long-term deconditioning status. In this perspective, benefit is not automatically achieved through high-technology interventions and pharmacological management alone. This study have shown that a short-term, supervised, exercise-based CR is feasible, safe and effective in elderly patients after TAVI, as well as after traditional surgery, and after LVAD implantation. An early CR programme enhances independence, mobility and functional capacity and should be encouraged in these subjects.

An early and intensive CR, based on physical activity and counselling, resulted to be safe and effective also in high risk patients after AMI, both in the short and in the long period. Indeed, a significant improvement in functional capacity in the short term - independent from the basal ventricular function or glucometabolic status - and a high adherence to therapy and to lifestyle modifications in the long term were achieved. Despite the high risk profile of these patients, this produced a favourable effect on cardiac and total mortality.

Keywords: cardiac rehabilitation, preventive cardiology, exercise capacity, six minute walking test, cardiopulmonary exercise test, outcome, transcatheter aortic valve implantation, left ventricular assist device, myocardial infarction.

Introduction

Despite the favourable effects of new therapeutic approaches during the acute phase of cardiac diseases and consequent favourable short-term outcomes, post-acute management and long term prognosis still remain unsatisfactory. Indeed cardiac diseases are still the leading causes of death in industrialized countries. They also induce considerable harm to survivors and often lead to severe and irreversible physical and neurological disabilities.

Cardiac rehabilitation (CR) is defined as "a multifaceted and multidisciplinary intervention witch aim to limit the adverse physiological and psychological effects of cardiac illness, to reduce morbidity and mortality, and to enhance the patient's psychosocial and vocational status".[1,2] Its beneficial effects are established for the vast majority of cardiac patients and it is universally considered an important aspect of secondary prevention.[3,4] Referral for CR is a class I indication (useful and effective) in most contemporary clinical practice guidelines, including those for ST-segment elevation myocardial infarction (MI),[5] unstable angina/non-ST-segment elevation MI,[6] coronary artery bypass graft (CABG) surgery,[7] valvular heart disease,[8] heart failure,[9] peripheral arterial disease.[10]

Contemporary cardiac rehabilitation can be divided into three phases. Each phase aims to facilitate recovery and to prevent further cardiovascular disease. Phase I, or inpatient phase, is initiated while the patient is still in the acute care hospital. It consists of early progressive mobilization of the stable cardiac patient to the level of activity required to perform simple household tasks. The shorter hospital stay with modern cardiology makes it difficult to conduct formal inpatient education and training programs. Thus inpatient cardiac rehabilitation programs are mostly limited to early mobilization to make self care possible by discharge, and brief counselling about the nature of the illness, the treatment, risk factors management and follow-up planning. In most countries, among which the USA, phase II is a supervised ambulatory outpatient program of 3 to 6 months duration which consists of outpatient monitored exercise and aggressive risk factor reduction. In Europe residential programs of 2 to 4 weeks duration are offered. In Italy both these realities coexist: lower risk patients usually are referred to out-patients programs and higher risk ones are referred to residential programs. This phase is managed in specialized centres by a multidisciplinary team comprehending cardiologists, physiotherapists, psychologists, nutritionists. Phase III is a lifetime maintenance phase in which physical fitness and additional risk-factor reduction are emphasized. It consists of home-or gymnasium-based exercise with the goal of continuing the risk factor modification and exercise program learned during phase II.[11]

Historical perspectives. The relative importance of physical activity for patients with so-called "disorders of the chest" was noted some 200 years ago. In 1772, Heberden published a report describing a six-month exercise program consisting of 30 minutes of daily sawing activity for one of his male patients who had a diagnosed chest disorder.[12] Parry, in 1799, independently noted the beneficial effects of physical activity in his patients who suffered from chest pain.[13] Although these reports were written long before any formal recognition or definition of coronary artery disease, undoubtedly some of these patients had experienced anginal disease or myocardial infarctions. This initial, apparently positive attitude toward physical activity was all but forgotten by the time Herrich, in 1912, gave his original clinical description of an acute MI.[14] Expressed concern regarding physical exertion and the increased risk of ventricular aneurysm rupture or heightened arterial hypoxemia precipitated the adoption of a conservative treatment approach in which patients were kept at bed rest for six to eight weeks post-MI. Pharmacological management of cardiac patients was limited. The agents

8

most commonly used were digitalis and nitroglycerin. The traditional medical management of physical inactivity for coronary patients was reinforced in the 1930s by two physicians, Mallory and White.[14] They found that the necrotic myocardial region transformed into scar tissue after about six weeks. Therefore, they advised a minimum of three weeks in bed for patients with even the smallest MI.[14] Continued limited physical activity was prescribed after patient hospital discharge. Stair climbing often was prohibited in some cases for up to a year. During this so-called convalescent period, the patient's tendency to become an invalid was enhanced. Follow-up medical management gave little advice to patients regarding functional cardiac capacity, stress management, or education about the disability and its limitations. Frequently, patients did not return to work and soon were considered as nonproductive members of society. Research during the first three decades of the twentieth century focused mainly on better methods of diagnosing and classifying cardiac disorders and simple testing for "circulatory efficiency".[15] Little emphasis was placed on the actual development or evaluation of the rehabilitation program.

By the late 1930s, many members of the labour force were retired on disability because of cardiac problems. The New York State Employment Service, concerned about the growing numbers of men on disability, decided to investigate the situation. A survey identified that 80% of the individuals receiving disability were coronary patients who had not returned to their jobs. Furthermore, only 10% had attempted either to retrain for another job or seek a different position in their company. In 1940, the New York State Employment Service asked the New York Heart Association to assist in evaluating cardiac workers to determine the level of activity the cardiac patient could perform safely. This request eventually led to the establishment of the Work Classification Unit or Work Evaluation Unit.[16] Cardiac work evaluation units were located in teaching hospitals, rehabilitation centres, and

community hospitals. Patients were referred by private physicians and employers and from institutions
and vocational agencies. At the unit, patients were evaluated for their physical and psychological capacity for work. Cardiologists performed laboratory tests, resting ECGs, and a Masters Step Test. Most evaluations took three weeks to complete and, after a team conference, recommendations were made to the referring party. No formal exercise program was included or prescribed for the patients. Thus, the cardiac work evaluation unit was an early approach to what we know today as cardiac rehabilitation.[16] Criticism grew, however, in the 1950s over the small numbers of patients being referred and the methods used to classify coronary disability. This situation caused fragmentation of evaluation and care of these patients. Gradually, the effectiveness and success of the units dwindled.

In 1952, Levine and Lown openly questioned the need for enforced bed rest and prolonged inactivity after an MI. Based on work performed in a Boston hospital during the 1940s and spurred by the manpower needs during World War II, they helped liberalize the attitudes among physicians regarding the need for rigid restrictions of activity. From their work, they concluded that long-continued bed rest "decreases functional capacity, saps morale, and provokes complications".[17] Their report caught the attention of many and raised numerous clinical questions about the management of cardiovascular disease. At the Thirteenth Scientific Session of the American Heart Association (AHA) in Chicago in 1953, the noted physician Louis Katz told the medical community that "physicians must be ready to discard old dogma when they are proven false and accept new knowledge".[18] The need to continue research on physical activity and to assimilate this new information into the practice scheme for the cardiac patient was emphasized. Turell and Hellerstein urged physicians to provide a more positive philosophy and a more comprehensive approach in treating cardiac patients.[19] The application of work physiology principles was stressed. They recommended a graded step program (a prototype to contemporary cardiac rehabilitation) based on established energy requirements of physical activity and patient exercise tolerance with continual evaluation of cardiovascular function. Thus, the prevailing theme of this period was clinical research on physical activity and its relationship to coronary artery disease. The strength of the new research provided visible evidence to a doubting medical society. Dwight Eisenhower, then President of the United States, suffered a heart attack in office. His physician was the noted Paul Dudley White, a man strongly committed to the positive effects of exercise. He prescribed graded levels of exercise, including swimming, walking, and golf, for his celebrated patient. This regimen was viewed by many physicians as reckless and inappropriate, especially given the patient's eminence. The result turned out to be so positive for President Eisenhower that he created the President's Youth Fitness Council, later to be renamed the President's Fitness Council by President Kennedy.[16]

By the 1960s, numerous studies demonstrated that early activity after an MI safely negates the adverse effects associated with prolonged bed rest. Saltin et al[20] reported that the functional capacity of normal subjects confined to bed for three weeks decreased approximately 33%. Equally important was his finding that an appropriate equal time of training was necessary to restore the subjects to their prebed-rest condition. After three months of twice-daily rigorous exercise programs, all patients exceeded their control states. Inpatient cardiac rehabilitation became more formalized in the sixties primarily through the efforts of Wenger[21] and Zohman,[22] and Bruce[23] in the fifties. The adopted programs instituted early supervised reconditioning during the acute post-MI phase while the patient was still in the Coronary Care Unit (CCU) and during the post-acute phase while the patient was in the step-down unit. The protocol of Wenger et al consisted of a 14-step program of progressively increasing physical activity levels with emphasis in three areas: graded physical exercises, activities of daily living, and educational activities.[21] The program usually was initiated in the CCU after the patient's clinical condition was stable. Physical activities at this stage required low-level oxygen demand. They included self-care and supervised active and passive range of motion exercises; progressive ambulation was added shortly thereafter. Patient and family education programs paralleled the graded physical activities. This structured plan greatly assisted the patient toward discharge and an early return to normal living. Zohman's program provided exercise using an equicaloric technique that matched the level of energy expenditure with exercise of equal caloric value.[22] The exercises were monitored by radiotelemetry, and energy costs were measured as a check on the rehabilitation activities. The favourable outcome of these structured programs encouraged the development of other similar programs around the USA. Soon, other hospitals also were experiencing the positive economic implications of early intervention. These included a hastened recovery time and decreased hospital stay; improved functional status at the time of discharge; and in turn, an earlier return to work.

By the end of the 1960s, Hellerstein encouraged by the results of his inpatient program, boldly chose to incorporate physical exercise into a follow-up program after hospital discharge. A formalized study was conducted involving 200 post-MI patients at the Cleveland YMCA and later at the local Jewish Community Center.[24] Hellerstein was criticized severely by his peers for his innovative but risky approach. The study clearly demonstrated that cardiac patients could benefit physiologically from regular progressive exercise and enjoy improved psychological confidence without a negative effect on either mortality or morbidity.[24] The success of this medically supervised program offered a new dimension, the outpatient program, to cardiac rehabilitation. As a result of the work of Hellerstein, Wenger, Zohman, and others, the concept of progressive supervised activity for the post-MI patient and the post-surgical patient has taken its rightful role in the practice of medical therapeutics.

Nowadays, despite the role of CR having been extensively documented, endorsed and promoted by a number of health care organizations and their position statements for the comprehensive secondary prevention of cardiovascular events, its use remains still rather limited in Europe and in the rest of the world.[25]

Aim. The aim of this PhD research was to examine some aspects still little known, or unknown at all, in the CR field. In particular, the research aimed to evaluate safety and efficacy of a structured, exercise-based, CR in specific cohorts of patients: after transcatheter aortic valve implantation (TAVI), after left ventricular assist device (LVAD) implantation, and early after (within 2 weeks) an acute myocardial infarction (AMI) in high risk subjects.

CR after TAVI. Due to the significant increase in the life span, nowadays degenerative-calcific aortic stenosis (AS) is the most common acquired valvular heart disease in the developed countries, affecting 2-7% of the population aged over 65 years.[8]

Once symptoms occur in severe AS, the prognosis is very poor without treatment with a mortality rate up to 50-60% after 2 years; surgical aortic valve replacement (sAVR) is currently the gold standard treatment for these patients[26] but about 30% of them are declined for surgery because of their high or prohibitive surgical risk.[27]

Transcatheter aortic-valve implantation (TAVI) is an innovative procedure, in which a bioprosthetic valve is inserted through a catheter and implanted within the diseased native aortic valve; at the moment, two models with substantial clinical data are available: the balloon-expandable Edwards Sapien™ and the self-expanding Medtronic CoreValve™.[28]

Since 2002, when the procedure was first performed,[29] there has been a rapid growth in its utilization throughout the world and now data from large

European observational registries - reporting both improved procedural success and mid-term survival - are available.[30,31] After results from the randomized Placement of AoRTic TraNscathetER Valves (PARTNER) trials, TAVI represents now the standard of care for extremely high risk or 'inoperable' patients and it is a valid alternative to surgery for selected high-risk but 'operable' patients with symptomatic AS.[32,33]

All patients after TAVI, because of their age and primary compromised conditions, are natural candidates for referral to exercise based CR; despite this, until now no data have been available about the safety and the efficacy of a comprehensive rehabilitative period in these subjects.

CR after LVAD implantation. In the last decade there was an expanding application of left ventricular assist devices in end-stage chronic heart failure patients, due to a shortage of donor organs combined with the efficacy of these mechanical circulatory supports.[34] The modern devices assist the left ventricle by means of a rotary pump applied on the left ventricle apex and generating a continuous axial flow from the apex of the left ventricle to the descending aorta. They can be applied both as temporary support (bridge to transplantation) or as permanent treatment in selected patients not suitable to heart transplantation. The positive effect of LVAD on left ventricular function (LV) include marked reduction in LV systolic and diastolic pressures, leading to reverse LV remodelling, a normalized pressure volume relation, and myocyte recovery, with improved contractile function. As a matter of fact LVAD recipients demonstrate improvement in exercise tolerance and non cardiac organ function.[35,36] However many of the studies in the literature regarding exercise capacity after LVAD were conducted on pulsatile machines - a type of LVAD the use of which is almost abandoned today – and relatively late after implantation (at least 3 to 7 months).[37,38]

Little is known about feasibility, safety and efficacy of a structure, exercise training in the early phase after LVAD implantation.[39]

Early CR after AMI in high risk patients. In coronary artery disease (CAD) patients exercise-based CR has lots of valuable effects: it improves symptoms, functional capacity, metabolic and psychological status, reducing both morbidity and mortality.[40-42] Recently, Martin et al.[43] among 5886 individuals who had undergone CR after an acute MI showed, in the completers, the lowest mortality and hospitalization rates as long as the fewest emergency room visits versus non completers. Furthermore, a strong dose–response relationship has also been demonstrated between the number of CR sessions and long-term outcomes with a lower risks of death and MI at 4 years.[44]

Even though maximal benefit of CR derives from early initiation of exercise (as early as 1 week after MI hospital discharge),[45] most of the rehabilitative programs begin too late after the acute event (more than one month). Furthermore the studies available in the literature regarding an early beginning of a structured physical activity after an acute MI were conducted in the pre-trombolitic era[46] or consider low risk, outpatients, cohorts.[47]

Methods

Patients. All patients (78 TAVI, mean age 82.1±3.6 years, 42 LVAD, 63.4 ± 7.4 years, and 376 AMI, 64.4±12.3 years) were referred to the Institute Codivilla-Putti (in Cortina d'Ampezzo, BL, Italy), in the period 2008-2013, for a two week, in-hospital, CR training and comprehensive risk factors interventions early after the acute event (within two weeks TAVI and AMI, within two months after LVAD implantation). TAVI and AMI patients were submitted by an unique centre (University Hospital of Padova), LVAD patients were referred by four different institutions (Padova, n=18, 43%, Udine, n=14, 33%, Siena, n=7, 16%, Bologna, n=3, 7%). Demography, medical history and conventional risk factors, physical examination and treatment data were recorded for all the patients; routine biochemical analyses - including haematic crasis, hepatic enzymes, serum creatinine, hemocoagulative pattern, lipid determination, glycated haemoglobin A1c (HbA1c) - were obtained on admission; a 2-D echocardiogram was performed before discharge. Functional capacity was assessed by a six-minute walking test (6MWT) on admission and at discharge and by a cardiopulmonary exercise test (CPET) at discharge, when clinically feasible. Safety (incidence of fatal events during in-hospital stay and complications requiring transfer to advanced medical unit) and effectiveness (changes in the functional capacity in the short term in all patients and adherence to therapy, to proposed lifestyle modifications and impact on prognosis in AMI patients) were considered.

CR after TAVI. TAVI patients (Edwards[TM] trans-apical n=16, 20%, Edwards[TM] trans-femoral n=47, 60%, Corevalve[TM] n=15, 20%) were compared with 80 consecutive peer patients who were admitted for CR in the same period after surgical aortic valve replacement (sAVR). All sAVR patients had received a biological prosthesis.

CR after LVAD. LVAD patients underwent the assist device implantation (Jarvik-2000 Flowmaker® 33, 78%, Berlin Heart Incor® 2, 4%, Heart Ware® 7, 16%) due to end-stage chronic heart failure (CHF). Shortly before intervention they often were in terminal conditions, they needed intensive inotropic support and usually had been bedridden for quite a long period. As a matter of fact, these patients began the programme in extremely poor general conditions. During CR stay, the device rotation speed was maintained unmodified, as initially set by the cardiac surgery team to allow maximum support while avoiding suction events (range 10000-11000 rpm, corresponding to a nominal device output at rest of 4 to 5 l/min). LVAD patients were compared with 47 coeval advanced CHF patients who were admitted for CR in the same period after an acute heart failure event. In order to assess cardiac autonomic function in the early phase after axial-flow LVAD implantation, heart rate variability (HRV) was also evaluated in 24 patients (those with atrial fibrillation, or rhythm mainly induced by a pace-maker, or with diabetes mellitus were excluded). The following HRV time-domain parameters were evaluated by the means of a 24h ECG Holter (Del Mar-Reynolds Impresario Holter Analysis System, vers. 2.8.0024): mean and minimum heart rate, standard deviation of all normal RR intervals (SDNN), square root of the mean square differences of successive NN intervals (RMSSD), standard deviation of the 5-min average of NN intervals (SDANN), proportion of successive beats with differences in NN intervals >50ms (pNN50), average of the standard deviations of all NN intervals for each 5-minute segments (SDNNindex) and HRV Triangular Index. The HRV parameters were evaluated both on the whole 24-h recording and subdivided by day and night.

CR after AMI. All patients had an angiography-documented CAD and 84.8% had received a percutaneous revascularization treatment in at least one vessel. They were selected by the submitting centre to our programme if they had a complicated AMI (cardiogenic shock or pulmonary edema, cardiac arrest, complex ventricular arrhythmias), an incomplete revascularization (because of clinical decision, unfavorable coronary anatomy or technical failure), or had at least 3 cardiovascular risk factors. Low risk patients followed an out-patient CR programme in another centre and were excluded from this study. Coronary artery bypass grafting, echo- or cardiac MRI-documented intracavitary thrombosis, extreme thinning or suspected rupture of the ventricular wall and/or intra-myocardial bleeding were exclusion criteria as well. In order to evaluate the influence of a reduced left ventricular ejection fraction (LVEF) on the rehabilitative process, the population was divided into 2 groups according to a 40% LVEF cut-off at enrolment. Moreover, in 326 patients a glucometabolic characterization was obtained by means of a standard oral glucose tolerance test (OGTT, 75 g anhydrous glucose in 200 ml water[48]) in patients without known diabetes. The test was performed during the 2nd week of stay in the rehabilitation centre, usually during the 3rd week after the acute event. The classification of the glucometabolic state was made according to the American Diabetes Association Criteria 2008:[49]

- Normal Glucose Tolerance (NGT) was defined as Fasting plasma glucose (FPG)<100 mg/dl (5.6 mmol/L) and glycaemia at the second hour after OGTT (OGTT-2h) <140 mg/dl (7.8 mmol/L);
- Impaired Fasting Glycaemia (IFG) as FPG ≥100 mg/dL (5.6 mmol/L) but <126 mg/dl (7.0 mmol/L);
- Impaired Glucose Tolerance (IGT) as OGTT-2h ≥140 mg/dl (7.8 mmol/L) but <200 mg/dl (11.1 mmol/L);

- Newly detected Diabetes Mellitus (DM) as either FPG ≥126 mg/dl (7.0 mmol/L) or OGTT-2h ≥200 mg/dl (11.1 mmol/L).

A prediabetic condition was defined when IFG and/or IGT was present. After OGTT administration 3 groups could be identified in the AMI cohort: NGT, prediabetics and diabetics (known or newly detected).

Rehabilitation programme. In all patients the training protocol consisted of a low/medium intensity exercise protocol developed in 3 sets of exercises, 6 days a week: 30 min of respiratory workout, followed by an aerobic session on a cyclette (or on an arm-ergometer for those patients who were not able to cycle) in the morning and, in the afternoon, 30 min of callisthenic exercises. Each session was supervised by a physician and a physiotherapist and all patients were ECG monitored by a telemetry system. Aerobic training was performed using a constant work rate modality without exceeding 70% of the maximal predicted peak heart rate (HR) for each patient.[50] Each aerobic session lasted 10 minutes at the beginning, with a 5 minutes progressive increase to reach a 30 min target; the exercise prescription and evaluation of exercise intensity was carefully derived from the subjective rating of perceived exertion, using a category ratio Borg scale.[50] Individual and group counselling meetings, psychological and nutritional evaluation were also performed for all patients.

Autonomy evaluation. The Barthel index (BI) was used as an autonomy index in TAVI and LVAD cohorts. The BI uses a scale of 0–100 to rate the degree of independence in activities of daily living, where 0 is total dependence and 100 is total independence.[51,52] This index was obtained from standardised interviews by nurses at entry and at discharge.

Six minute walking test. The walking test was performed in an indoor unobstructed 30 m long corridor, according to the American Thoracic Society recommendations.[53] All patients were informed in a standardized manner of the purpose and method of the test before the test was performed. They were instructed to walk the corridor from one end to the other at their own pace, as many time as possible, in the permitted time. They were advised on the possibility of slowing down the pace and stopping or resting as needed to resume walking as soon as they felt they were able to do so. After six minute had elapsed patients were instructed to stop walking and the total distance was measured. The test was supervised by a physical therapist or a physician who encouraged the patients in a standardized fashion at regular intervals.[53]

Cardiopulmonary exercise test. The cardiopulmonary exercise test (CPET) was performed at the end of the rehabilitation period, usually on the day before discharge. The test was performed in the late mornings, at least 3 hours after a light meal, on a computer driven cycle ergometer (*Cardiovit CS-200 Ergo-Spiro, Schiller AG, Baar, CH ; Ergoselect 100 ergometer, Ergoline GmbH, Bitz, D*). A progressive ramp protocol of 6 to 10 W/min was used, after a 1 min adaptation and warm-up period at 0 Watts, until subjective exhaustion or appearance of the clinical and electrocardiographic criteria for termination of a stress test (progressive angina, ST segment depression ≥ 2 mm, symptomatic hypotension, hypertension, major arrhytmias).[54] Expired gas was collected by means of a tightly fitting face mask and continuously analyzed during the exercise test (*Schiller Ganshor CS-200 Power Cube*). The oxygen consumption (VO_2) at the peak of the exercise was expressed relative to body weight (ml/Kg/min); in the text the term VO_2 max is referred to peak VO_2; the anaerobic threshold (AT) was determined non-invasively using a dual-method approach (both the ventilatory equivalents and the V-slope methods); the peak exercise capacity was expressed in Watt as maximum sustained workload (Watt-max). The peak respiratory exchange ratio (RER max) was calculated as VCO_2/VO_2 at the peak of the exercise.[55] Ventilatory response to exercise (minute ventilation per unit of carbon dioxide production, VE/VCO_2 slope) was calculated with the slope calculation option of the spreadsheet software package. The slope of circulatory efficiency (VO_2/W slope) from rest to peak exercise in millilitres of oxygen uptake per watt of external work was determined by linear regression analysis. The oxygen uptake efficiency slope (OUES), defined as the constant a in the linear relationship between $\log_{10}VE$ (l/min) to VO_2 (ml/min), was calculated over the entire duration of the incremental exercise ($VO_2 = a \times \log_{10}VE + b$). The kinetics of VO_2 recovery after exercise ($T_{1/2}VO_2$, defined as the time in seconds elapsing during the recovery phase before oxygen uptake equals half of the increase in VO_2 between peak effort and baseline VO_2) was also analyzed.[55]

Follow up. In AMI patients rate of death, hospitalizations, smoke cessation, physical activity and adherence to pharmacological treatment were recorded at follow up (up to 5 years, median 2 years).

Each patient or first degree relatives were contacted by phone by a physician. Because 11 patients (2.9%) were lost at follow-up, final population resulted to be 365 subjects. Informations on all-cause and cardiac mortality and occurrence of major adverse cardiovascular events (MACE) (new AMI, new revascularization, heart failure or stroke) were collected. As secondary end-points adherence to therapy and life-style changes (smoking cessation and physical activity defined as more than at least 3 aerobic exercise sessions per week, of 30 min each) were assessed.

Statistical Analysis. Continuous variables normally distributed (Kolmogorov-Smirnov and Shapiro Wilk tests for data normality were used) were expressed as a mean ± standard deviation and compared using an unpaired t-test, otherwise variables were expressed with median and interquartile range (IQR) and compared using a Wilcoxon-Mann-Withney test. Categorical variables were expressed as frequencies and percentages and were compared between groups by a chi-squared test. The relationships between continuous variables were evaluated by Pearson's correlation coefficient. Survival curves were calculated by the Kaplan-Meier method and groups were compared with a log-rank test. A Cox regression multivariate analysis was also performed to determine the influence of different factors (age>65 years, EF<40%, diabetes, ST elevation MI, chronic renal failure, atrial fibrillation, left bundle branch block) on all cause mortality. All reported probability values are two-tailed and the significance level was set at 0.05. Statistical analyses were performed using SPSS 18 software package (SPSS Inc, Chicago, IL,USA).

Results

CR after TAVI [56,57]

Clinical characteristics are shown in table 1. The two groups (TAVI and sAVR) were similar in terms of age, gender, mean time from the valve prosthesis implantation to the CR beginning and the mean stay in the CR. Furthermore, no significant differences were found in the prevalence of hypertension, diabetes or pre-diabetes, metabolic syndrome, coronary artery disease and myocardial infarction history, atrial fibrillation, left ventricular ejection fraction, haemoglobin (Hb) values. Most patients were in NYHA class III (90%) in both groups. As expected, the TAVI group showed more comorbidities and a higher prevalence of left bundle branch block and new pace maker implantation but with a similar, extremely low, drop out rate compared to sAVR group (only one case per group had to be transferred to an acute hospital for non fatal complications). In both groups non significant change in weight was observed in the short term.

A higher percentage of TAVI patients took double antiplatelet therapy (77% vs 3%, p<0.01) while a higher percentage of sAVR ones was on anticoagulant therapy (69% vs 30%, p<0.01). The use of amiodarone was more frequent in the sAVR group (43% vs 16%, p=0.01). No significant differences were found between groups in the use of beta-blockers, as well as calcium antagonist, angiotensin-converting enzyme inhibitor, angiotensin II receptor antagonist, diuretics and statins use (Table 1).

Autonomy evaluation. Even though, in absolute terms, sAVR patients reached a higher level of autonomy after CR than the TAVI ones (BI at discharge 98.3±4.3 vs 90.3±17.2, p=0.01), at the end of the CR period, all patients enhanced independence and mobility (mean BI increment 9.9±12.6, p<0.01) and were able to walk at least with the assistance of a stick (Table 2).

Change in the six minute walking test. There was a significant increase in the six minute walk distance at discharge compared with baseline (Δ6MWT in the entire population: 66.5±52.0 m, p<0.001), with no significant differences in Δ6MWT between groups (Table 2, Figure 1).

Cardiopulmonary exercise test. A smaller percentage of patients were able to perform the CPET in the TAVI than in the sAVR group; in those patients who were able to complete the test, exercise capacity at the end of the rehabilitation programme did not differ significantly between groups (mean W-max 35.2±16.2 vs 42.3±12.2 W, p=0.06; mean peak-VO$_2$ 12.5±3.6 vs 13.9±2.7 ml/kg/min, p=0.01; Table 2, Figure 1). No significant differences were found between groups in the HR at exercise peak, in the rate-pressure product, in the VO$_2$ and HR at anaerobic threshold, in the peak respiratory exchange ratio and in the minute ventilation/carbon dioxide output slope (Table 2). A correlation was found between the peak VO$_2$ and the distance walked at 6MWT on discharge (r= 0.42 , p<0.01; Figure 2).

Table 1. CR after TAVI: clinical features

	TAVI n=78	sAVR n=80	All n=158	p
Clinical characteristics				
Age (yrs)	83.3±3.6	81.0±3.1	82.1±3.6	0.06
Age [min-max]	[77-89]	[76-88]	[76-89]	
Male sex (%)	31.7	50.0	40.0	0.10
Hypertension (%)	95.1	94.1	94.7	0.84
Diabetes (%)	24.4	23.5	24.0	0.93
Pre-diabetes (%)	37.2	40.0	38.5	0.80
Metabolic Syndrome (%)	63.4	79.4	70.7	0.13
Coronary artery disease (%)	65.1	65.7	65.4	0.95
Previous MI (%)	17.1	14.7	16.0	0.78
Previous PCI (%)	31.7	2.9	18.7	<0.01
Previous CABG (%)	14.6	2.9	9.3	0.08
Vascular disease (%)	26.8	17.6	22.7	0.34
Pulmonary disease (%)	30.2	2.9	17.3	<0.01
Renal Failure (%)	27.9	14.3	21.8	0.14
Cancer (%)	19.5	11.8	16.0	0.36
LBBB (%)	47.5	17.6	33.8	<0.01
Newly implanted Pace Maker (%)	12.2	2.9	8.0	0.14
Atrial Fibrillation (%)	25.6	25.7	25.6	0.98
BMI (kg/m^2)	24.7±3.7	26.0±3.8	25.3±3.8	0.14
LVEF (%)	55.9±11.3	57.2±8.5	56.7±9.8	0.55
NYHA	2.93±0.26	2.97±0.17	2.95±0.22	0.40
Haemoglobin at entry (g/dL)	10.3±0.9	10.2±1.0	10.2±0.9	0.33
Stay in CR (days)	16.6±4.7	16.1±2.9	16.4±3.9	0.58
Time implant-rehab (days)	13.3±12.5	14.2±10.8	13.7±11.7	0.55
Drop out (n/tot) (%)	1/78 (1.3)	1/80 (1.3)	2/158 (1.3)	0.89
Causes	Arrhythmias	Acute Abdomen		
Medication (%)				
Aspirin	95.3	74.3	85.9	<0.01
Clopidogrel	76.7	2.9	43.6	<0.01
Warfarin	27.9	68.6	46.2	<0.01
ß-blockers	51.2	65.7	57.7	0.21
Calcium antagonist	25.6	11.4	19.2	0.11
Amiodarone	16,3	42,9	28,2	0.01
ACE-I	51.2	51.4	51.3	0.98
AT-II ant	23.3	14.3	19.2	0.31
Diuretics	79.1	80.0	79.5	0.91
Statins	76.7	62.9	70.5	0.18

TAVI= transcatheter aortic valve implantation; sAVR= surgical aortic valve replacement; CABG= coronary artery bypass graft; PCI= percutaneous coronary intervention; LBBB= Left Bundle Branch Block; BMI= body mass index; LVEF=Left ventricular ejection fraction; NYHA= New York Heart Association; ACE-I = angiotensin-converting enzyme inhibitor; AT-II ant = angiotensin II receptor antagonist. Renal failure= at least moderate reduction in glomerular filtration rate (30-59 ml/min/1.73 m2)

Table 2. CR after TAVI: autonomy evaluation and functional status assessment

	TAVI n=78	sAVR n=80	All n=158	p
Barthel Index (BI)				
At entry BI	80.9±24.3	87.6±14.5	84.1±20.5	0.16
At discharge BI	90.3±17.2	98.3±4.3	94.0±13.4	0.01
Δ BI	9.3±12.3	10.6±13.2	9.9±12.6	0.67
6MWT (n/tot) (%)	64/78 (82)	74/80 (92)	138/158 (87)	
Basal (mt)	240.8±94.9	259.6±98.2	250.6±96.1	0.51
Pre-discharge (mt)	272.7±107.8	294.2±100.8	283.6±104.0	0.42
Δ6MWT (mt)	60.4±46.4	72.3±57.3	66.5±52.0	0.45
CPET (n/tot) (%)	48/78 (61)	60/80 (75)	108/158 (68)	
Max workload (W)	35.2±16.2	42.3±12.2	39.6±14.5	0.06
Peak-VO_2 (ml/Kg/min)	12.5±3.6	13.9±2.7	13.4±3.1	0.16
Peak-VO_2 (% predicted)	70.3±18.4	73.4±17.9	72.2±17.9	0.61
HR max (beat/min)	96.7±21.0	100.5±19.4	98.9±19.9	0.56
HR max (% predicted)	70.3±14.8	73.4±14.8	72.1±14.7	0.53
RPP (mmHg·beat/min)	12913±4615	13793±4238	13436±4353	0.55
AT HR (beat/min)	85.3±17.8	91.4±18.6	89.1±18.3	0.38
AT VO_2 (ml/Kg/min)	10.8±2.9	14.7±9.7	13.3±8.0	0.20
RER max	1.04±0.1	1.08±0.1	1.06±0.1	0.22
VE/VCO_2 slope	30.0±6.4	29.8±4.4	29.9±5.1	0.89

TAVI= transcatheter aortic valve implantation; sAVR= surgical aortic valve replacement; 6MWT= six minute walking test; Δ6MWT= change in the 6 min walking test (mean calculated only in those patients who performed both the baseline and pre-discharge test); CPET= cardiopulmonary exercise testing; Peak-VO_2= peak O_2 consumption; HR max= maximal heart rate; AT HR= anaerobic threshold heart rate; RPP= rate-pressure product; AT VO_2= anaerobic threshold O_2 consumption; RER max= maximal respiratory exchange ratio; VE/VCO_2 slope= minute ventilation/carbon dioxide output slope.

Figure 1. CR after TAVI. Change in the distance walked at 6MWT and peak VO2 according to TAVI and sAVR groups

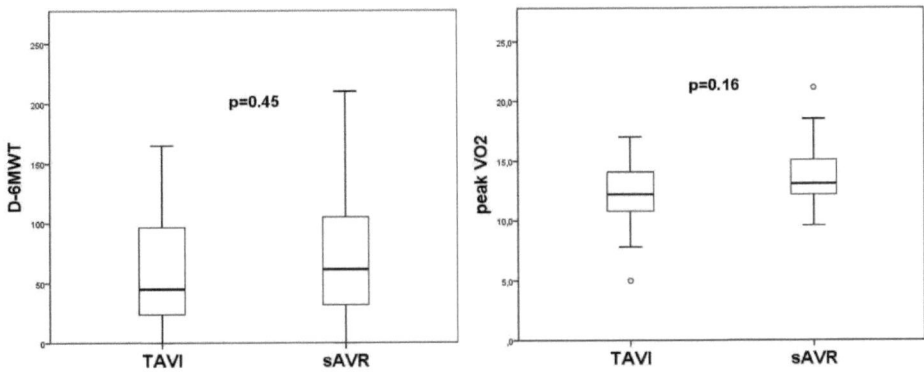

Figure 2. CR after TAVI. Correlation between the peak VO_2 at CPET and the distance walked at 6MWT on discharge

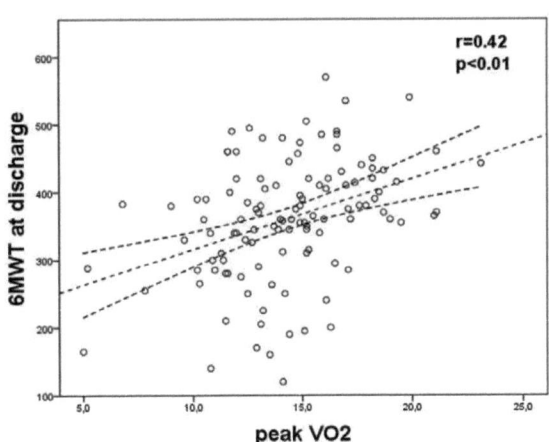

CR after LVAD [58-62]

Both LVAD and CHF patients were in extremely poor general conditions. As a result of the selection criteria, the two groups presented similar clinical features (age, gender, the time interval from the index event - device implantation or acute heart failure - were comparable (Table 3). Left ventricular ejection fraction (LVEF) was particularly low in both groups, even if in LVAD group it was slightly lower. As expected, INTERMACS class (level of limitation according to profiles defined by the Interagency Registry for Mechanically Assisted Circulatory Support) was significantly lower in LVAD than in CHF cases (Table 3). All patients were anemic (mean Hb values at entry 9.2±1.5 g/dl, minimum 6.0 g/dL – maximum 11.6 g/dL, at discharge 10.2±1.5 g/dL, minimum 6.6 g/dL – maximum 12.8 g/dL). During the CR stay (mean 18,6 ± 8,0 days, min 5 - max 40 days) 5 patients dropped out of the programme due to complications requiring transferral in acute care hospitals (3 cases of major bleedings, 1 sternal wound dehiscence, 1 ictus cerebri).

Exercise capacity. In the completers, at the end of the CR period all patients enhanced independence and mobility (mean BI increment 11.9±10.5, $p<0.01$) and were able to walk at least with the assistance of a stick. A 6MWT could be performed in 76% of LVAD patients with a mean increment in the distance walked of 83 ± 36 mt ($p<0.05$). The mean distance walked at 6MWT at entry was 272 ± 55 mt (min 168 – max 345 mt), at discharge 354 ± 64 mt (min 230 – max 490 mt).

At the cardiopulmonary exercise test (Table 3), both LVAD and CHF patients were able to sustain a rather poor workload: CHF patients reached a W-max of 56.6 ± 18.2 W, while LVAD patients reached an even lower value of 36.3 ± 9.0 W ($p<0.001$). Peak-VO$_2$ was slightly more depressed in LVAD patients than in reference CHF cases, but the difference did not reach statistical significance, neither in absolute terms nor as a percentage of the expected values. When the peak-VO_2 reached by the patients was adjusted for the haemoglobin levels, the peak oxygen uptake resulted to be slightly, but not significantly greater in LVAD than in CHF patients. The VO_2 at anaerobic threshold (AT) was similar between the two groups, but LVAD patients reached AT at a significantly lower workload than CHF cases (Table 3).

There was a tendency towards a lower oxygen uptake efficiency slope (OUES) in LVAD than in CHF patients, but the difference did not reach statistical significance. The slope of circulatory efficiency (VO_2/W slope) was similar between the two groups of patients. The ventilatory efficiency (VE/VCO_2 slope) was also similar in the two groups (Table 3).

During the recovery phase from ergometric stress, in the group of LVAD patients the kinetics of oxygen uptake recovery ($T_{1/2}VO_2$) was superior (p=0.04). No significant correlation was found between $T_{1/2}VO_2$ and peak-VO_2 or Hb levels both for CHF patients (respectively: rho -0.144, p=0.568; rho -0.381, p=0.119) and LVAD-supported patients (respectively: rho 0.117, p=0.643; rho -0.111, p=0.660; rho 0.022, p=0.931).

Heart rate at the peak of exercise test was higher in LVAD compared to CHF patients, while heart rates at 1 and 2 minutes after the end of exercise were similar (Table 3).

Cardiac autonomic function. The mean and the minimum heart rate (HR) recorded during the 24-h ECG Holter were significantly higher in LVAD patients compared to controls (Table 4). Heart rate variability (HRV) parameters estimating overall (SDNN, Triangular Index) and slow oscillation (SDANN) autonomic activity were significantly depressed in LVAD patients in the early phase after device implantation (Table 4). Similar results were found also in the separate analysis of the day and the night periods (Table 5). No significant variations were found among the groups concerning HRV parameters estimating high frequency oscillations (RMSSD, pNN50).

In the analysis of circadian oscillations of HRV for individual patients, LVAD patients did not show significant day/night variations of any HRV parameter; the same was also evident for the group of CHF patients not supported by LVAD.

Table 3. CR after LVAD. Main clinical and CPET parameters

	LVAD	CHF	p
Age (years)	63.4 ± 7.4	64.6 ± 5.3	0.51
Male (%)	81.0	83.0	0.73
Time from index event	38.5 ± 18.3	30.3 ± 20.8	0.13
LVEF (%)	20.3 ± 6.3	24.4 ± 4.0	0.01
INTERMACS class	2.5 ± 0.8	4.2 ± 0.5	<0.001
Hb levels (g/dl)	10.8 ± 1.1	12.4 ± 2.0	<0.01
CPET parameters			
W-max, W	36.3 ± 9.0	56.6 ± 18.2	<0.001
Peak-VO_2, ml/kg/min	12.5 ± 3.0	13.6 ± 2.9	0.16
Peak-VO_2 percentage of expected (%)	48.8 ± 13.9	54.2 ± 15.3	0.19
Peak-VO_2 corrected by Hb, ml/kg/min	19.5 ± 4.2	18.1 ± 4.4	0.25
AT-VO_2, ml/kg/min	10.4 ± 2.5	10.9 ± 2.2	0.50
AT-Watt, W	25.2 ± 9.6	39.9 ± 13.2	<0.001
VO_2/W slope	11.5 ± 3.8	12.0 ± 2.0	0.63
OUES, ml/min	1124.2 ± 226.3	1280.2 ± 391.1	0.08
VE/VCO_2 slope	32.2 ± 3.6	33.9 ± 8.5	0.34
$T_{1/2}VO_2$, sec	212.5 ± 62.5	261.1 ± 80.2	0.04
RER-max	1.07 ± 0.08	1.12 ± 0.10	0.06
Peak HR, bpm	112.4 ± 18.8	101.5 ± 16.1	0.03
HR-1, bpm	100.8 ± 14.0	93.4 ± 13.3	0.06
HR-2, bpm	93.4 ± 12.2	86.5 ± 13.6	0.06

LVAD: patients with left ventricular assist device; CHF: patients with chronic heart failure; p: level of statistical significance; LVEF: left ventricular ejection fraction; INTERMACS class: level of limitation according to profiles defined by the Interagency Registry for Mechanically Assisted Circulatory Support; Hb: haemoglobin; CPET: cardiopulmonary exercise test; W-max: maximum sustained workload; peak-VO_2: peak oxygen uptake; AT-VO_2: oxygen uptake at anaerobic threshold; AT-Watt: Watts at anaerobic threshold; VO_2/W slope: slope of circulatory efficiency (oxygen uptake/power output slope); OUES: oxygen uptake efficiency slope; VE/VCO_2: ventilatory equivalent of carbon dioxide; $T_{1/2}VO_2$: kinetics of VO_2 recovery after exercise; RER-max: peak respiratory exchange ratio; HR: heart rate; HR-1 and HR-2: heart rate 1 and 2 min after end of exercise.

Table 4. CR after LVAD. HRV parameters

	LVAD	CHF	p
HRV parameters			
Mean HR, bpm	94.6 ± 16.4	68.4 ± 10.9	<0.001
Minimum HR, bpm	79.5 ± 8.5	55.9 ± 10.1	<0.001
pNN50, %	6.9 ± 7.2	8.1 ± 9.5	0.61
SDNN	53.7 ± 18.3	91.9 ± 37.1	<0.01
RMSSD	40.7 ± 29.7	45.0 ± 36.2	0.66
Triangular Index	6.6 ± 2.5	11.7 ± 3.9	<0.001
SDNN Index	23.1 ± 10.7	33.5 ± 19.3	0.06
SDANN	42.7 ± 12.4	81.1 ± 34.2	<0.001

HRV: heart rate variability; LVAD: patients with left ventricular assist device; CHF: congestive heart failure patients; HR: heart rate; pNN50: proportion of successive beats with differences in NN intervals >50ms; SDNN: standard deviation of all normal RR intervals; RMSSD: square root of the mean square differences of successive NN intervals; SDANN: standard deviation of the 5-min average of NN intervals.

Table 5. CR after LVAD. HRV parameters: day/night (D/N)

	LVAD	p (D/N)	CHF	p (D/N)
SDNN day	48.8 ± 16.4	0.91	85.2 ± 36.1	0.82
SDNN night	49.2 ± 19.5		86.3 ± 39.3	
RMSSD day	38.3 ± 27.0	0.16	46.9 ± 42.9	0.28
RMSSD night	42.1 ± 30.3		41.3 ± 24.8	
SDNN Index day	21.9 ± 10.4	0.04	34.3 ± 22.9	0.79
SDNN Index night	24.2 ± 10.0		33.6 ± 17.0	
SDANN day	37.5 ± 12.6	0.72	73.0 ± 27.9	0.73
SDANN night	36.3 ± 13.1		74.4 ± 38.7	

See Table 4 for abbreviations

CR after AMI [63,64]

Baseline characteristics of the study population are reported in table 6 and 7. On the whole 87% of the patients had a complicated AMI and 47% were incompletely revascularized. The median length of in-hospital stay during the acute phase before transferring to CR unit was 14 days (IQR 10,18 days). At admission at the CR unit, 84% of patients showed a NYHA functional class II or III. No significant differences in terms of age, sex, length of stay in the rehabilitative unit, rate of smokers, percentage of incomplete revascularization and prevalence of metabolic syndrome were observed between those with LVEF<40% and with LVEF>40%. Lower LVEF group showed higher rate of previous AMI (25.3% vs 16.1%, p = 0.04), lower incidence of STEMI, greater degree of anemia, and longer in-hospital stay during the acute phase (Table 6). Diabetic patients were older and, as expected, had worse clinical conditions (Table 7). After administration of an OGTT, a prediabetic status was found in 54% of patients without known diabetes. Prediabetic patients had intermediate clinical characteristic between the normal glucose tolerance (NGT) group and diabetics (Table 7).

Overall, no fatal events occurred during the CR stay (median 15 days, IQR 13,16 days). Four patients (1,1%) dropped out of the programme because of non-fatal complications: 2 subjects with unstable, refractory angina and 2 with persistent arrhythmias (1 with complete AV block and 1 with non-sustained ventricular tachycardia). At the end of the CR programme, the vast majority of the patients were on aspirin, statins, beta-blockers and ACE inhibitors, irrespective to basal LVEF (Table 6).

Exercise capacity. At the end of the rehabilitative period, in all patients a significant improvement in functional status, as measured by the 6MWT, was observed (Table 8-9). Individuals with LVEF<40% walked a shorter distance throughout the CR period, but no differences in term of functional recovery were found compared with patients with higher LVEF (Table 8). Exercise capacity as assessed by CPET was significantly poorer in the subjects with LVEF<40%. As expected, these patients achieved lower maximal workload, rate-pressure product and oxygen consumption both at the peak exercise and at the anaerobic threshold, also the VE/VCO2 slope resulted higher (Table 8). Diabetics had the absolute lowest exercise capacity compared to prediabetics and NGT patients. Exercise performance in prediabetics was intermediate compared to the other groups (Table 9, Figure 3). Furthermore, a prediabetic status resulted an independent predictor of the 6MWT at discharge and the peak oxygen consumption achieved at CPET (B -0,220, p<0,01).

Outcome. *Behavioral habits.* Active smoking habits at the time of the AMI were recorded in 32.1%. Among these subjects, 77% definitively quitted at the follow up. In the whole population, 73% reported to continue regular physical activity. This group showed a lower rate of MACE when compared to sedentary subjects (10.8% vs 22.8%, p 0.02), despite no difference in age between the groups (63.76±12.4 years vs 62.0±12.4 years, p=ns).

Adherence to therapy. At the follow-up, high adherence to therapy was registered: 96.4% of the patients were on aspirin; 85.2% beta-blockers; 95.6% statins and 89.0% ACE-Inhibitors or AT II antagonists (Table 6).

Mortality and major cardiovascular events. Cardiac and all cause mortality resulted 5.0% and 8.0 % at 1 year and 8.0 % and 13.0 % at 5 years, respectively and resulted higher in older people, in those with lower LVEF, and in diabetics (Figure 4-5, Table 10). At multivariate analysis age>65 years, (regression coefficient B=-0.64, p=0.03), EF<40% (B= 0.86, p<0.01) and presence of diabetes (B= -0.73, p=0.01) resulted independent predictors of adverse outcome

Table 6. CR after AMI. Clinical features according to residual LVEF

	LVEF < 40 n=99	LVEF > 40 n=277	All n=376	p
Clinical characteristics				
Age (yrs)	66.1±11.6	63.7±12.5	64.4±12.3	0.11
Male sex (%)	78.8	76.9	77.4	0.69
STEMI (%)	51.0	67.1	62.7	<0.01
Vessels with critical lesions (%)				
1	28.9	33.3	32.2	
2	23.7	29.3	27.9	0.20
3	47.4	36.2	39.1	
Vessels treated (%)				
1	48.0	54.0	52.4	
2	19.4	24.3	23.0	0.10
3	10.2	9.1	9.4	
Incomplete revascularization (%)	52.5	44.4	46.5	0.16
Hypertension (%)	79.8	75.3	76.5	0.38
Diabetes (%)	43.4	23.0	28.2	<0.01
Pre-diabetes (%)	30.1	42.0	39.0	0.06
Metabolic Syndrome (%)	72.7	69.4	70.3	0.56
Previous MI (%)	25.3	16.1	18.5	0.04
Previous PTCA (%)	14.3	13.9	14.0	0.91
Previous CABG (%)	12.1	6.9	8.3	0.10
Vascular disease (%)	21.2	6.5	10.4	<0.01
Pulmonary disease (%)	10.1	3.7	5.4	0.01
Renal Failure (%)	14.1	5.9	8.1	0.01
Atrial Fibrillation (%)	9.1	5.1	6.2	0.16
Current smoker at MI onset (%)	33.3	31.7	32.1	0.77
NYHA class II/III (%)	45.5/47.5	53.3/22.3	51.2/29.0	<0.01
LVEF (%)	33.8±4.9	51.7±6.9	47.0±10.2	<0.01
BMI (kg/m^2)	27.2±5.5	27.4±4.3	27.4±4.6	0.69
Haemoglobin at entry (g/dL)	11.5±1.6	12.4±1.5	12.2±1.6	<0.01
Stay in CR (days)	15 (13,17)	14 (13,16)	15 (13,16)	0.02
Time to rehab (days)	16 (13,25)	13 (10,17)	14 (10,18)	<0.01
Drop out (n) (%)	0 (0.0)	4 (1.4)	4 (1.1)	0.23
Medication (%)				
Aspirin	98.9	97.8	98.1/96.4*	0.48
Clopidogrel	90.4	96.0	94.6	0.04
ß-blockers	89.4	89.0	89.1/85.2*	0.92
ACE-I	78.7	83.9	82.6/71.3*	0.26
AT-II ant	14.9	11.7	12.5/16.4*	0.42
Statins	98.9	97.8	98.1/95.6*	0.49

LVEF=Left ventricular ejection fraction; STEMI=ST elevation myocardial infarction; MI=myocardial infarction; PTCA: percutaneous transluminal coronary angioplasty; CABG: coronary artery bypass graft; NYHA= New York Heart Association; BMI= body mass index; ACE-I = angiotensin-converting enzyme inhibitor; AT-II ant = angiotensin II receptor antagonist. Renal failure= at least moderate reduction in glomerular filtration rate (30-59 ml/min/1.73 m2). *(At discharge/follow up).

Table 7. CR after AMI. Clinical features according to glucometabolic status

	NGT n=107	Pre-diabetes n=127	Diabetes n=92	All n=326	p
Clinical characteristics					
Age (yrs)	59.7±12.8	64.5±12.1	67.0±10.2	63.6±12.1	<0.01
Male sex (%)	80.4	78.7	75.0	78.2	0.65
STEMI (%)	75.7	63.0	51.6	64.0	<0.01
Vessels with critical lesions (%)					
1	42.9	36.5	15.6	32.7	<0.01
3	23.8	35.7	57.8	38.0	
Vessels treated (%)					
1	63.6	51.6	45.1	53.7	0.11
3	5.6	10.3	11.0	9.0	
Incomplete revascularization (%)	39.3	39.4	63.0	46.0	<0.01
Hypertension (%)	68.2	76.8	88.2	77.0	<0.01
Metabolic Syndrome (%)	45.8	84.9	93.4	73.5	<0.01
Previous MI (%)	15.2	14.3	28.3	18.6	0.04
Previous PTCA (%)	11.5	10.3	19.6	13.4	0.11
Previous CABG (%)	6.7	5.6	14.1	8.4	0.06
Vascular disease (%)	6.5	3.2	23.9	10.2	<0.01
Pulmonary disease (%)	2.9	4.8	8.7	5.3	0.18
Renal Failure (%)	5.7	7.3	12.0	8.1	0.25
Atrial Fibrillation (%)	1.9	7.9	7.6	5.9	0.11
Current smoker at MI onset (%)	38.3	31.5	27.1	32.6	0.24
NYHA class II (%)	47.7	64.6	35.6	50.9	<0.01
III (%)	12.1	19.7	56.7	27.5	<0.01
LVEF (%)	48.4±8.9	48.6±10.5	44.3±10.4	47.3±10.1	<0.01
BMI (kg/m^2)	26.7±3.6	27.2±4.2	29.0±5.4	27.4±4.3	<0.01
Haemoglobin at entry (g/dL)	12.3±1.6	12.3±1.6	12.0±1.4	12.2±1.5	0.26
Stay in CR (days)	14 (13,16)	15 (13,15)	15 (13,17)	15 (13,16)	0.01
Time to rehab (days)	13 (10,18)	13 (9,18)	14 (11,19)	14 (10,18)	0.55
Medication (%)					
Aspirin	98.1	98.4	98.9	98.4	0.92
Clopidogrel	92.5	95.3	96.6	94.7	0.43
ß-blockers	91.6	88.2	90.8	90.0	0.66
ACE-I	88.8	81.9	75.9	82.6	0.06
AT-II ant	8.4	14.2	17.2	13.1	0.17
Statins	98.1	98.4	98.9	98.4	0.92
Insulin therapy	0.0	0.0	61.5	17.2	<0.01
Oral hypoglycemic agents	0.0	0.0	33.0	9.2	<0.01

NGT=Normal glucose tolerance; STEMI=ST elevation myocardial infarction; MI=myocardial infarction; PTCA: percutaneous transluminal coronary angioplasty; CABG: coronary artery bypass graft; LVEF=Left ventricular ejection fraction; NYHA= New York Heart Association; BMI= body mass index; ACE-I = angiotensin-converting enzyme inhibitor; AT-II ant = angiotensin II receptor antagonist. Renal failure= at least moderate reduction in glomerular filtration rate (30-59 ml/min/1.73 m2).

Table 8. CR after AMI. Functional status assessment according to residual LVEF

	LVEF < 40 n=99	LVEF > 40 n=277	All n=376	p
6MWT				
Basal (mt)	356.5±135.7	424.2±122.5	407.5±129.1	< 0.01
Pre-discharge (mt)	411.3±134.0	491.3±122.1	471.3±129.7	<0.01
Δ6MWT (mt)	65.9±62.9	72.2±53.2	70.7±55.7	0.37
CPET				
Max workload (W)	62.7±22.3	83.1±31.2	78.2±30.6	<0.01
Peak-VO$_2$ (ml/Kg/min)	15.2±3.9	18.2±5.2	17.5±5.1	<0.01
Peak-VO$_2$ (% predicted)	62.6±18.2	72.2±18.8	69.9±19.1	<0.01
HR max (beat/min)	107.6±16.8	109.2±18.7	108.8±18.2	0.52
HR max (% predicted)	70.3±10.4	69.1±10.6	69.4±10.6	0.38
RPP (mmHg·beat/min)	14664±4208	16777±4698	16265±4666	<0.01
AT HR (beat/min)	94.5±12.5	90.7±14.7	91.6±14.3	0.05
AT VO$_2$ (ml/Kg/min)	12.1±2.5	14.0±6.3	13.5±5.6	0.02
RER max	1.1±0.1	1.1±0.1	1.1±0.1	0.77
VE/VCO$_2$ slope	28.8±4.9	26.3±4.4	26.8±4.6	<0.01

6MWT= six minute walking test; Δ6MWT= change in the 6 min walking test; CPET= cardiopulmonary exercise testing; Peak-VO$_2$= peak O$_2$ consumption; HR max= maximal heart rate; AT HR= anaerobic threshold heart rate; RPP= rate-pressure product; AT VO$_2$= anaerobic threshold O$_2$ consumption; RER max= maximal respiratory exchange ratio; VE/VCO$_2$ slope= minute ventilation/carbon dioxide output slope.

Table 9. CR after AMI. Functional status assessment according to glucometabolic status

	NGT n=107	Pre-diabetes n=127	Diabetes n=92	All n=326	p
6MWT					
Basal (mt)	464.2±118.4	421.7±111.1	344.2±121.8	414.9±125.0	<0.01
Pre-discharge (mt)	532.9±117.6	488.5±110.4	404.4±125.2	479.9±127.1	<0.01
Δ6MWT (mt)	74.2±59.6	63.8±45.9	74.1±62.1	70.0±55.3	0.29
CPET					
Max workload (W)	88.8±35.5	80.0±27.2	66.3±24.0	79.6±30.9	<0.01
Peak-VO$_2$ (ml/Kg/min)	19.4±5.5	17.9±4.8	15.3±4.1	17.8±5.1	<0.01
Peak-VO$_2$ (% predicted)	72.8±18.2	73.0±20.1	64.2±18.4	70.7±19.3	<0.01
HR max (beat/min)	111.5±18.2	110.0±18.6	105.2±17.4	109.3±18.3	0.07
HR max (% predicted)	69.7±10.3	69.9±10.6	68.8±11.3	69.6±10.7	0.78
RPP (mmHg·beat/min)	17400±4723	16715±4604	14676±4325	16465±4686	<0.01
AT HR (beat/min)	93.0±13.3	91.3±14.0	91.0±17.0	91.8±14.5	0.64
AT VO$_2$ (ml/Kg/min)	14.5±3.8	13.3±3.4	12.0±2.9	13.4±3.6	<0.01
RER max	1.1±0.0	1.1±0.1	1.1±0.1	1.1±0.1	0.21
VE/VCO$_2$ slope	26.4±5.4	26.3±3.8	27.6±4.5	26.7±4.6	0.15

NGT=Normal glucose tolerance; 6MWT= six minute walking test; Δ6MWT= change in the 6 min walking test; CPET= cardiopulmonary exercise testing; Peak-VO$_2$= peak O$_2$ consumption; HR max= maximal heart rate; AT HR= anaerobic threshold heart rate; RPP= rate-pressure product; AT VO$_2$= anaerobic threshold O$_2$ consumption; RER max= maximal respiratory exchange ratio; VE/VCO$_2$ slope= minute ventilation/carbon dioxide output slope.

Figure 3. CR after AMI. Functional capacity according to glucometabolic status. Maximum work load (A) and peak VO$_2$ at CPET (B)

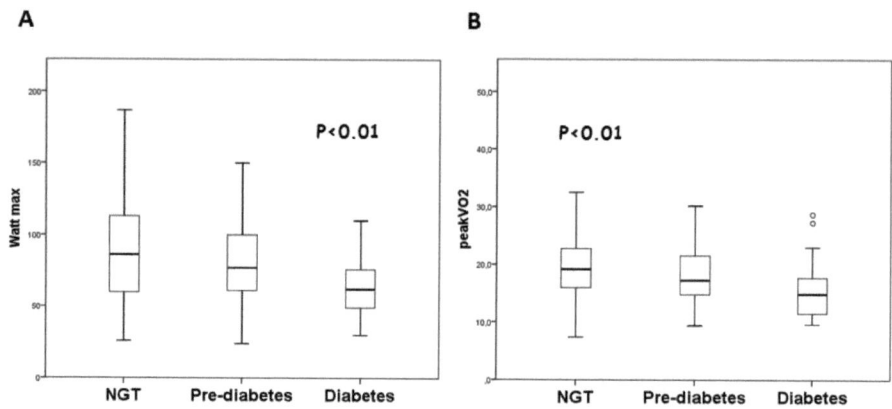

Table 10. CR after AMI. Events at follow up according to residual LVEF (unadjusted data)

Events (n) (%)	LVEF < 40 n=95	LVEF > 40 n=270	Age > 65 n=177	Age < 65 n=188	All n=365	p*	p±
All-cause death	15 (15.8)	13 (4.8)	25 (14.1)	3 (1.6)	28 (7.7)	0.01	<0.01
Cardiac death	13 (13.7)	5 (1.9)	15 (8.5)	3 (1.6)	18 (4.9)	<0.01	0.02
MACE	30 (31.6)	42 (15.6)	46 (26.0)	26 (13.8)	72 (19.7)	0.01	0.04
Myocardial infarction	2 (2.5)	7 (2.7)	8 (5.3)	1 (0.5)	9 (2.7)	0.91	0.07
PTCA/CABG	3 (3.8)	18 (7.0)	11 (7.2)	10 (5.4)	21 (6.2)	0.29	0.48
Heart Failure	13 (16.3)	12 (4.7)	13 (8.6)	12 (6.5)	25 (7.4)	0.01	0.47
Stroke	1 (1.3)	6 (2.3)	6 (3.9)	1 (0.5)	7 (2.1)	0.55	0.03

* p between LVEF groups; ± p between age groups; MACE=Major Adverse Cardiovascular Events (Cardiac mortality, re-infarction, new PTCA/CABG, heart failure, stroke); LVEF=Left ventricular ejection fraction; PTCA: percutaneous transluminal coronary angioplasty; CABG: coronary artery bypass graft

Figure 4. CR after AMI. All cause-mortality according to age groups (A) and left ventricular ejection fraction (B)

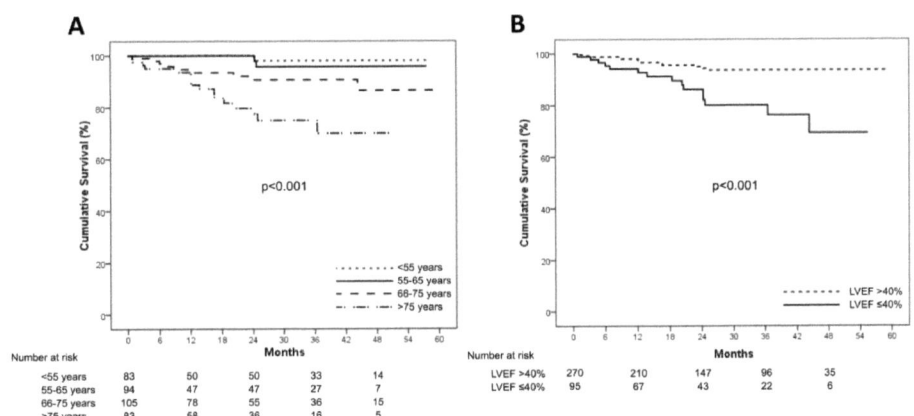

Figure 5. CR after AMI. Risk of major adverse cardiovascular events according to glucometabolic status

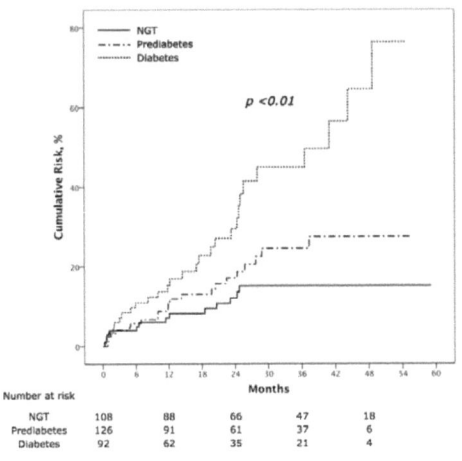

Discussion

CR after TAVI. This study demonstrates, for the first time, both safety and efficacy of an early, intensive, CR in very elderly patients after TAVI as well as after the traditional surgical aortic valve replacement. Actually, in spite of the training intensity, our structured CR programme resulted absolutely feasible with an extremely low drop-out rate and a satisfactory number of 6MWT performed in both groups. At the end of the rehabilitative period, all patients enhanced independence, mobility and functional capacity, all were able to walk at least with the assistance of a cane. As expected, compared to sAVR, a smaller percentage of TAVI patients was able to perform a 6MWT or a CPET because of their more compromised conditions; nevertheless, in those who were able, performances reached did not differ from the traditional surgery ones.

Cardiac rehabilitation is strongly recommended for patients after cardiac surgery,[2] particularly in very elderly people due to their age-dependent comorbidities and physical limitations. Despite this, octogenarians are rarely referred to CR programmes and very few studies have selectively investigated this subgroup of patients. Scant available data indicates that, in over 70s, the functional impairment assessed on admission considerably improved by means of CR, and that elderly patients gain a functional ability increase, not dissimilarly from younger ones.[65,66]

In our investigation, the CR programme started immediately after surgery (within the second week). Although in some European countries and in few Italian centres an early in-hospital CR is applied, in the majority of rehabilitative institutions patients are generally referred to an out-patient CR centre after a mean of 4 to 8 weeks post-surgery.[25,67] However, Macchi et al[68] showed that, in selected patients aged over 75 years who have undergone cardiac surgery, long-term rehabilitation outcomes are also favourable, and that an early (within the second week after the operation) rehabilitation programme can be as effective and safe as a late one (within the fourth week).

Even if sAVR remains the standard of care for most patients with symptomatic severe AS, TAVI has been increasingly recognized as a curative treatment choice. After the publication of several real-world registries and the pivotal PARTNER randomized trials, TAVI has become the standard of care for patients for whom surgical risk is prohibitive, and a reasonable alternative for selected operable patients with a high risk of either mortality or morbidity.[28]

Beyond improvement of life expectancy, an important goal of TAVI in older patients is to enhance their functional status. Apart from age and comorbidities, severe aortic stenosis represent a "per se" contraindication to physical activity so that patients usually arrive at the operation in a very deconditioned status.

In the literature available, very few data exist on the functional evaluation of patients after TAVI. Gotzmann et al[69] and Bagur et al[70] performed a 6MWT before and after TAVI (30 days and 6 months respectively) showing a significant increase in the mean distance walked. These findings, unrelated with any structured rehabilitation, are somehow not surprising as after intervention there is a reduction of the aortic gradient leading to left ventricular unloading and to an improvement in functional capacity.

To the best of our knowledge, no study has assessed the effect on an early, structured, CR programme on functional recovery after TAVI. Comparing two 6MWT (both performed after TAVI, pre and post-CR) we found a significant improvement in the short period (Δ6MWT: 60.4±46.4 mt, p<0.001); even if the absolute exercise capacity evaluated by 6MWT was quite low in the TAVI group, it was not significantly different from that found in the sAVR group (Table 2, Figure 1).

The 6MWT is a simple and reliable tool for the assessment of functional capacity in CR; it is also reproducible and is more reflective of activities of daily life than other tests.[71] Our data confirm the previously reported correlation between the distance walked in the 6MWT and the VO_2 achieved at peak exercise during a cycle ergometer test.[72,73] However, the data provided by the 6MWT should be considered complementary to the CPET; in fact in those patients capable of performing the test, the CPET can add important information without additional risks.[74]

We found a low functional capacity as assessed by CPET, both in the sAVR and in the TAVI group (Table 2). This could be explained partly by the aging process itself, partly by the disease and comorbidities that lead to prolonged inactivity. With aging, oxidative and inflammatory stress and perhaps apoptosis lead to molecular and cellular changes in skeletal muscle, extracellular matrix, vessel wall and intravascular compartment.[75] Another factor that could have worsened the exercise capacity is anemia. In our series a high prevalence of a mild grade of anemia was found, without significant differences between TAVI and sAVR (Haemoglobin at entry respectively: 10.3 ± 0.9 vs 10.2 ± 1.0g/dL, p=0.33). Reduced haemoglobin levels are rather frequent in CR and do not preclude functional recovery, as previously demonstrated in a study referring to various cardiac pathologies.[76] It is noteworthy that in those patients who were able to walk or cycle functional capacity was not significantly different between TAVI and sAVR patients. A possible explanation is that, although TAVI patients had more comorbidities than the controls, they underwent an indubitably less invasive procedure that could have accelerated the recovery process in the short period after the operation.

CR after LVAD. It is known that the implantation of a mechanical circulatory support in patients with advanced CHF leads to an improvement of hemodynamic parameters,[77,78] whose clinical effects are visible rather early after beginning of support.[79] However, scant data are present in the literature on effort tolerance and feasibility of an exercise training in patients in assistance by an axial-flow LVAD earlier than 2 months after implant, a period when patients are usually discharged to their homes.[80] Laoutaris et al,[81] in a very little cohort (14 patients), reported the efficacy of a structured exercise training when the program began at least 6 month after LVAD implantation. To our best knowledge, the present study, reporting the greatest number of axial-flow LVAD cases observed so far, demonstrate that a structured exercise training is feasible, safe and effective in the early phase of circulatory support. Indeed, considering the extremely high risk cohort of patients, a relatively low percentage of drop out was observed. In the completers, all patients at the end of the program enhanced their autonomy and improved their functional capacity as measured by 6MWT.

In spite of the short time elapsed since beginning circulatory assistance, a considerable percentage of patients, supported by LVAD due to refractory heart failure, were able to tolerate a sub-maximal stress test at the end of the short period of rehabilitation. This is an remarkable result, if we take into account that these patients were in extremely poor clinical conditions only a short time before, they had recently undergone major surgical stress and they had been bedridden for quite a long period. In spite of these constraints, LVAD patients were able to reach at CPET a peak-VO_2 similar to that of CHF patients in less compromised baseline clinical conditions; particularly, there was no difference between the two groups concerning the percentage of expected peak-VO_2, based on age, sex and body surface area. The peak-VO_2 in our LVAD patients was also similar to that reported by Dimopoulos et al,[82] that observed a much smaller number of axial-flow LVAD (7 cases) compared to 14 CHF cases. The working capacity of LVAD cases, expressed in terms of afforded workload (both maximum sustained workload and workload at anaerobic threshold), was anyway much poorer compared to the reference group of advanced CHF patients.

A parameter that showed a tendency towards slightly poorer values in LVAD cases was the oxygen uptake efficiency slope (OUES), whose values were approximately 12% lower than those observed in CHF cases. To our knowledge, this is the first report of the behaviour of OUES in LVAD assisted patients. OUES is an indicator of cardiovascular and peripheral factors that determine oxygen uptake, as well as of pulmonary factors that influence ventilatory response to exercise; it is linked to development of metabolic acidosis, physiological dead space and arterial carbon dioxide partial pressure. Differently from OUES, the ventilatory response to exercise (VE/VCO_2 slope, a parameter linked to the ventilation/perfusion mismatch, and to the occurrence of lactic acidosis and chemoreflex activity) showed a tendency towards better results in LVAD than in CHF patients. Anyway the differences of the reported parameters were small and showed no statistically significant difference among the two groups (possibly due to the low number of cases), so that only speculative considerations may be drawn. The slightly shallower slope of the VO_2/Watt slope and poorer OUES could suggest a still limited capacity of the LVAD patients (compared to the more stable CHF subjects) to adapt to the non-steady-state conditions of the ramp exercise. A reduced O_2 extraction by a low mass of exercising muscles and impaired skeletal muscle metabolism (due to physical deconditioning), jointly with the inability of LVAD to raise muscle blood flow appropriately to provide O_2 rapidly enough to satisfy muscle requirements (due to the almost fixed output of the device, in presence of low variations of peripheral resistances in untrained muscles), may explain the findings. On the other side, a decrease in pulmonary capillary pressure induced by the LVAD[83] could have led to a reduction of lung ventilation/perfusion mismatch, with the resultant small reduction in the VE/VCO_2 slope.

44

At the end of the exercise test, LVAD patients presented peak heart rates that were higher than those registered in CHF patients; in spite of this, heart rates slowed in the first two minutes of recovery, reaching values that were not dissimilar to those of CHF cases. These data are somehow different from what observed by Dimopoulos et al,[82] and could suggest a slightly quicker restoration phase in our LVAD supported cases; this behaviour is in accordance with the reduced $T_{1/2}VO_2$ in LVAD compared to CHF. The recovery kinetics of oxygen consumption following maximal exercise ($T_{1/2}$ of VO_2 recovery) is a reproducible parameter, that is usually reported not to be significantly affected by the exercise level achieved and to be directly correlated with the severity of the disease in CHF patients.[84] The tendency to a shorter $T_{1/2}VO_2$ observed in our LVAD patients may suggest a greater efficiency in the elimination of the accumulated oxygen debt, seemingly linked to the increased output given by the circulatory assistance.

LVAD patients were more anaemic compared to the group of CHF controls. Anaemia is known to reduce effort tolerance and peak oxygen uptake in patients with chronic heart failure,[85-87] as oxygen carrying capacity of the blood (mainly determined by the available Hb, and the $Hb-O_2$ saturation/dissociation curve) is one of the four major factors influencing oxygen uptake during physical effort, together with the central (cardiac) component, regional and local distribution of peripheral blood flow, and tissue capacity of O_2 extraction (capillary density, mitochondrial density and function, adequacy of perfusion, and tissue diffusion).[88] When peak-VO_2 was adjusted by Hb levels,[89] peak oxygen consumption of our LVAD patients resulted to be slightly (not significantly) greater than that of the reference group of CHF. Together with defective muscular mass and metabolic potential, anemia could have contributed to the persisting poor performance of LVAD patients.

It is known that in CHF patients, cardiac dysautonomia, as assessed by the analysis of heart rate variability (HRV), is associated with the degree of left ventricular dysfunction.[90,91] Theoretically, after LVAD implantation the increase of the circulatory output, accompanied by a restoration of beta-adrenergic density and responsiveness in cardiomyocites, in conjunction with reversal of the myocardial receptor downregulation, should progressively reduce cardiac sympathetic activation, improve neuroendocrine function and normalize overall autonomic system activity.[92-94] However, clinical studies on a possible recovery of cardiac autonomic function after implantation of a LVAD are controversial.[95,96] Our data show that in end-stage CHF patients early after a continuous-flow LVAD implantation, in spite of an amelioration of functional capacity, a profound autonomic derangement is still evident (even poorer than those found in the control group of advanced CHF patients). This findings could presumably explained both by a more advanced heart failure before device implantation and by the effects of a recent major surgery. Indeed, before the intervention, the patients subsequently implanted with LVAD were in terminal conditions and needed intensive inotropic support. Moreover, It is known that in many surgical interventions,[97,98] humoral factors and stress-induced activation of neural mechanisms of autonomic cardiovascular regulation are linked to an impairment of HRV that can persist for variable periods of time (up to one year).

CR after AMI. To our knowledge, this is the first study that has investigated, in a real world setting, the safety and efficacy of an early (within 2 weeks from the index event) and intensive (in hospital, 3 sessions daily, 6 days for week) exercise-based CR in high risk patients after AMI. Safety was demonstrated by the low dropout rate (only 1.1 %) and by the absence of major complications during the rehabilitation programme, despite the severe clinical profile of the patients at enrolment; efficacy by the significant improvement of

46

functional capacity in the short-term, irrespective from the basal ventricular function, and by the high adherence to therapy and to the proposed lifestyle modifications at follow up. Notably, the final net consequence in the long term might be a favorable effect on reduction of cardiac and total mortality, which indeed resulted low in our high risk population.

The safety of a structured exercise training has been widely documented in CAD patients, when the exercise programme, mostly extensive, started at least 1 month after the acute event. Vongvanich P. et al.[99] registered 4 non-fatal major events (3 cardiac arrests and 1 AMI), in a 9-years period with only one serious complication every 67.126 hours of exercise per patient. More recently, Pavy and colleagues,[100] analyzing data from 65 cardiac rehabilitation centers in France, confirmed the low rate of major cardiovascular events during rehabilitation: 1 event every 8484 stress tests or every 49.565 hours of exercise and 1.3 cardiac arrests per million hours of exercise. However, still very little is known about the safety of an aerobic training initiated soon after AMI. In 1982, Sivarajan et al.[46] demonstrated the safety and efficacy of an exercise programme started shortly after AMI (mean 4.5 days) and maintained for 3 months, on 135 patients compared to controls (61 patients), receiving conventional medical management. In this study, nevertheless, patients older than 70 years or with complicated AMI were excluded. More recently, Aamont et al.[47] evaluated the effect of an early start in exercise training in low risk patients after uncomplicated AMI (14 days after the event) compared with a delayed start control group (4 weeks after the event). This randomized study included a small number of patients: 20 subjects in the first group (60.9 ± 10.8 years old) and 19 in the second (57.7 ± 9.2 years old). Exercise training was completed without complications by all participants and the CPET showed improvement in functional capacity in both groups after CR, with no differences between them. Compared to these studies, our data first demonstrated that a structured, in-hospital, exercise training conducted under rigorous medical surveillance, without delay after the clinical stabilization, with a progressive intensity increase, is safe also in high risk patients after a complicated AMI.

The beneficial effects of exercise-based CR on functional capacity have been clearly documented in CAD patients.[101,102] In our study, at the end of the 2 week rehabilitative period, all patients increased the distance walked (mean 6MWT gain 70.67±55.7 m, p<0.05). Similar results have been reported elsewhere: in this case, however, patients were younger, at lower risk and followed an 8 weeks extensive CR programme.[103]

Importantly, in our study, functional recovery was independent from the basal LVEF and glucometabolic status: in fact, patients with LVEF<40% and diabetics, despite worse clinical characteristics and a lower absolute functional capacity at CPET, showed a functional recovery similar to the controls. After OGTT administration, a high prevalence of abnormal glucose metabolism was found (54%). As previously demonstrated,[73] our data confirmed that in prediabetics exercise capacity is better than diabetic but poorer than normoglicemic patients.

The most important aim of a comprehensive CR is to positively modify the risk factors cluster, in particular smoking and physical inactivity.[2,25]

In worldwide clinical records, the rate of smokers who quit definitively after an AMI varies from 28% to 75%.[104,105] In our analysis, the rate of smoke cessation at the follow up was 77%. These data confirms the importance of frequent and incisive counselling interventions, carried out by qualified professionals, supported by psychologists and supplemented by teaching materials. Interestingly, part of the advantage might be attributed to the particular timing of the educational intervention (immediately post AMI), when the patient is more prone to lifestyle changes, combined with the impossibility of smoking because of the hospitalization.

Seventy three per cent of our patients confirmed to continue regular aerobic activity for at least 30 minutes, 3 times a week. To this regard, it is noteworthy that physically active patients showed lower incidence of MACE compared to non- or less-active patients (10.8% vs 22.6%, p=0.02), independently from age, confirming the beneficial effects of physical exercise in post AMI patients.

According to the literature, data regarding adherence to prescribed therapies (aspirin, beta-blockers, ACE-I/ARB-II and statins) after AMI are discouraging. Approximately 20-50% of patients do not follow the pharmacological prescriptions and the drugs have been interrupted already in the first month after AMI, with subsequent serious impact on survival.[106] In our study more than 90% of patients continued to take the prescribed medications after 5 years. Adherence depends on many factors, but the doctor-patient relationship plays a crucial role and lack of time by health professionals often represents a serious obstacle for the realization of the indispensable "therapeutic alliance" between patients and care givers. In this scenario, a comprehensive CR may play a fundamental role by reinforcing the therapeutic suggestions provided during the acute phase of the disease.[41]

Favorable effects of CR on prognosis after AMI have been established.[42-44,101] This is the result of life-style interventions and of positive effect of physical activity on ventricular remodelling and on the residual LVEF.[107] A recent meta-analysis by Haykowsky et al.[45] on 1029 clinical trials confirmed that exercise training has beneficial effects on LV remodelling in clinically stable post-AMI patients, with the greatest benefits in increase of LVEF and decrease of LV end-systolic and end-diastolic volume. In a recent Italian survey on patients discharged from the intensive care units after AMI, all cause mortality at 30-day was 5.6% and 3.4% for ST elevation AMI and non ST elevation AMI patients, respectively.[108] In the United States, Coles et al.,[109] observed in 2007 a total mortality rates on post AMI unselected patients, of 8.9%, 16.4%, and 23.4%, at 3-month, 1-year, and 2-year, respectively, suggesting the need to enhance post-discharge management practices. Although it is difficult to compare populations with different clinical features and treated by different strategies, both all-cause and cardiac mortality in our study resulted low, especially considering the high risk profile of the population, suggesting the particular beneficial effects of our CR programme.

Limitations and future perspectives

These are observational, single centre, not randomized, studies. Since CR is today considered a class I recommendation, patient randomization could be difficult and perhaps not appropriate for ethical reasons.

The studies were conducted in an in-hospital setting, where the patients began the rehabilitative interventions early after the acute event and followed a relatively short period of intensive, exercise-based CR, under strict surveillance by a team including a physician. This kind of programme is still relatively uncommon in Europe and in the USA, where the majority of patients follow longer-term, lower-intensity, outpatient rehabilitation, often monitored only by physiotherapists. Whether the results of these studies are applicable to these programmes is unknown. Furthermore, the optimal type of training, as well as the optimal training frequency and intensity need further investigations.

Conclusions

Patients who underwent TAVI and LVAD implantation are characterized by a long-term deconditioning status. In this perspective, benefit is not automatically achieved through high-technology interventions and pharmacological management alone. This study have shown that a short-term, supervised, exercise-based CR is feasible, safe and effective in elderly patients after TAVI, as well as after traditional surgery, and after LVAD implantation. An early CR programme enhances independence, mobility and functional capacity and should be encouraged in these subjects.

An early and intensive CR, based on physical activity and counselling, resulted to be safe and effective also in high risk patients after AMI, both in the short and in the long period. Indeed, a significant improvement in functional capacity in the short term - independent from the basal ventricular function or glucometabolic status - and a high adherence to therapy and to lifestyle modifications in the long term were achieved. Despite the high risk profile of these patients, this produced a favourable effect on cardiac and total mortality.

Acknowledgements

I would like to thank the chief of the Preventive Cardiology and Rehabilitation Dr. Fabio Bellotto, my colleagues Dr. Leonida Compostella and Dr Tiziana Setzu, the managing director Dr. Massimo Miraglia and all the staff of the Institute Codivilla-Putti in Cortina d'Ampezzo. Last but not least my tutor Prof. Sabino Iliceto, inspiring this research program, and the University of Padua PhD program director Prof. Gaetano Thiene.

References

1. Wenger NK. Current status of cardiac rehabilitation. J Am Coll Cardiol 2008; 51: 1619–31.
2. Piepoli MF, Corra` U, Benzer W, et al. Secondary prevention through cardiac rehabilitation: physical activity counselling and exercise training. Eur Heart J 2010; 31:1967–1976
3. AHA; ACC; National Heart, Lung, and Blood Institute, et al. AHA/ACC guidelines for secondary prevention for patients with coronary and other atherosclerotic vascular disease: 2006 update endorsed by the National Heart, Lung, and Blood Institute. J Am Coll Cardiol 2006;47:2130-9.
4. Smith SC, Benjamin EJ, Bonow RO, et al. AHA/ACCF Secondary Prevention and Risk Reduction Therapy for Patients With Coronary and Other Atherosclerotic Vascular Disease: 2011 Update. Circulation 2011;124:2458-2473
5. O'Gara PT, Kushner FG, Ascheim DD, et al. 2013 ACCF/AHA guideline for the management of ST-elevation myocardial infarction: a report of the American College of Cardiology Foundation/American Heart Association Task Force on Practice Guidelines. J Am Coll Cardiol 2013; 61:e78-140
6. Anderson JL, Adams CD, Antman EM, et al. 2012 ACCF/AHA focused update incorporated into the ACCF/AHA 2007 guidelines for the management of patients with unstable angina/non-ST-elevation myocardial infarction: a report of the American College of Cardiology Foundation/American Heart Association Task Force on Practice Guidelines. Circulation 2013; 127:e663-828
7. Hillis LD, Smith PK, Anderson JL et al. 2011 ACCF/AHA Guideline for Coronary Artery Bypass Graft Surgery. A report of the American

College of Cardiology Foundation/American Heart Association Task Force on Practice Guidelines. J Am Coll Cardiol 2011; 58:e123-210

8. Vahanian A, Alfieri O, Andreotti F, et al. Guidelines for the Management of Valvular Heart Disease (version 2012). Eur Heart J 2012; 33, 2451–2496

9. McMurray JJ, Adamopoulos S, Anker SD, et al. ESC Guidelines for the diagnosis and treatment of acute and chronic heart failure 2012: The Task Force for the Diagnosis and Treatment of Acute and Chronic Heart Failure 2012 of the European Society of Cardiology. Eur Heart J 2012; 33:1787-847

10. Hirsch AT, Haskal ZJ, Hertzer NR, et al. ACC/AHA 2005 Practice Guidelines for the management of patients with peripheral arterial disease (lower extremity, renal, mesenteric, and abdominal aortic): a collaborative report from the American Association for Vascular Surgery/Society for Vascular Surgery, Society for Cardiovascular Angiography and Interventions, Society for Vascular Medicine and Biology, Society of Interventional Radiology, and the ACC/AHA Task Force on Practice Guidelines. Circulation 2006; 113:e463-654

11. Niebauer J (Editor). Cardiac rehabilitation manual. Springer 2011. ISBN 978-1-84882-793-6

12. Heberden W. Some accounts of a disorder of the chest. Med Trans Coll Physician 1772; 2:59

13. Parry CH. An Inquiry into the Symptoms and Causes of Syncope Anginosa Commonly Called Angina Pectoris. London, England, Caldwell and Davis, 1799

14. Mallory GK, White PD, Salcedo-Salger J. The speed of healing of myocardial infarction: A study of the pathological anatomy of seventy-two cases. Am Heart J 1939; 18:647-671

15. Masters AM, Oppenheimer ET. A simple exercise tolerance test for circulatory efficiency with standard tables for normal individuals. Am J Med Sci 177:223, 1929

16. Certo CM. History of cardiac rehabilitation. Phys Ther 1985; 65:1793-1795

17. Levine SA, Lown B. Armchair treatment of acute coronary thrombosis. JAMA 1952; 148:1365

18. Katz LN. Symposium: Unsettled clinical questions in the management of cardiovascular disease. Circulation 1953; 18: 430-450

19. Turell D, Hellerstein H. Evaluation of cardiac function in relation to specific physical activities following recovery from acute myocardial infarction. Prog Cardiovasc Dis 1958; 1:237

20. Saltin B, Bloomquist G, Mitchell JH, et al. Response to exercise after bedrest and after training. Circulation 1968; 38:1-78

21. Wenger N. The use of exercise in the rehabilitation of patients after myocardial infarction. J SC Med Assoc 1969; 65:66-68

22. Zohman L, Tobis JS. A rehabilitation program for inpatients with recent myocardial infarction. Arch Phys Med Rehabil 1968; 49:443

23. Bruce RA. Evaluation of functional capacity in patients with cardiovascular disease. Geriatrics 1957; 12:317

24. Hellerstein H. Exercise therapy in coronary disease. Bull NY Acad Med 1968; 44:1028-1047

25. Bjarnason-Wehrens B, McGee H, Zwisler AD, et al. Cardiac rehabilitation in Europe: results from the European Cardiac Rehabilitation Inventory Survey. Eur J Cardiovasc Prev Rehabil 2010; 17:410-8

26. Varadarajan P, Kapoor N, Bansal RC, et al. Survival in elderly patients with severe aortic stenosis is dramatically improved by aortic

valve replacement: Results from a cohort of 277 patients aged ≥80 years. Euro J Cardiothorac Surg 2006; 30: 722 – 727

27.   Florath I, Albert A, Boening A, et al. Aortic valve replacement in octogenarians: identification of high-risk patients. Eur J Cardiothorac Surg 2010; 37:1304-10

28.   Genereux P, Head SJ, Wood D, et al. Transcatheter aortic valve implantation 10 year anniversary: review of current evidence and clinical implications. Eur Heart J 2012; 33, 2388–2400

29.   Cribier A, Eltchaninoff H, Bash A, et al. Percutaneous transcatheter implantation of an aortic valve prosthesis for calcific aortic stenosis: first human case description. Circulation 2002;106:3006-8

30.   Eltchaninoff H, Prat A, Gilard M, et al. Transcatheter aortic valve implantation: Early results of the FRANCE (FRench Aortic National CoreValve and Edwards) Registry. Eur Heart J 2011; 32: 191-197

31.   Ussia GP, Barbanti M, Petronio AS, et al. Transcatheter aortic valve implantation: 3-year outcomes of selfexpanding CoreValve prosthesis. Eur Heart J 2012;33:969–976

32.   Leon MB, Smith CR, Mack M, et al. Transcatheter aortic-valve implantation for aortic stenosis in patients who cannot undergo surgery. N Engl J Med 2010; 363: 1597 – 1607

33.   Smith CR, Leon MB, Mack M, et al. Transcatheter versus Surgical Aortic-Valve Replacement in High-Risk Patients. N Engl J Med 2011; 364:2187–2198

34.   Kirklin JK, Naftel DC, Kormos RL, et al. The fourth INTERMACS annual report: 4,000 implants and counting. J Heart Lung Transplant 2012; 31:117-126

35.   Bank AJ, Mir SH, Nguyen DQ, et al. Effects of left ventricular assist devices on outcomes in patients undergoing heart transplantation. Ann Thorac Surg 2000; 69:1369-74

36.   Jacquet L,Vancaenegem O, Pasquet A, et al. Exercise capacity in patients supported with rotary blood pumps is improved by a spontaneous increase of pump flow at constant pump speed and by a rise in native cardiac output. Artif Organs 2011;35: 682-90.

37.   Guan Y, Karkhanis T, Wang S, et al. Physiologic benefits of pulsatile perfusion during mechanical circulatory support for the treatment of acute and chronic heart failure in adults. Artif Organs 2010; 34:529–36

38.   Haft J, Armstrong W, Dyke DB, et al. Hemodynamic and exercise performance with pulsatile and continuous-flow left ventricular assist devices. Circulation 2007;116(Suppl. 1):I-8–I-15

39.   Corrà U, Pistono M, Mezzani A, et al. Cardiovascular prevention and rehabilitation for patients with ventricular assist device from exercise therapy to long-term therapy. Part I: Exercise therapy. Monaldi Arch Chest Dis 2011; 76:27-32

40.   Taylor RS, Brown A, Ebrahim S, et al. Exercise-based rehabilitation for patients with coronary heart disease: systematic review and metaanalysis of randomized controlled trials. Am J Med. 2004;116:682–92.

41.   Giannuzzi P, Temporelli PL, Marchioli R, et al; GOSPEL Investigators. Global secondary prevention strategies to limit event recurrence after myocardial infarction: results of the GOSPEL study, a multicenter, randomized controlled trial from the Italian Cardiac Rehabilitation Network. Arch Intern Med 2008; 168:2194 –2204.

42.   Goel K, Lennon RJ, Tilbury RT, Squires RW, Thomas RJ. Impact of Cardiac Rehabilitation on Mortality and Cardiovascular Events After Percutaneous Coronary Intervention in the Community. Circulation 2011;123:2344-2352.

43.   Martin BJ, Hauer T, Arena R, et al. Cardiac Rehabilitation Attendance and Outcomes in Coronary Artery Disease Patients. Circulation 2012; 126:677-687

44.   Hammill BG, Curtis LH, Schulman KA, Whellan DJ. Relationship Between Cardiac Rehabilitation and Long-Term Risks of Death and Myocardial Infarction Among Elderly Medicare Beneficiaries. Circulation 2010; 121:63-70

45.   Haykowsky MJ, Liang Y, Pechter D, Jones LW, McAlister FA, Clark AM. A meta-analysis of the effect of exercise training on left ventricular remodeling in heart failure patients: the benefit depends on the type of training performed. J Am Coll Cardiol 2007; 49:2329 –2336.

46.   Sivarajan ES, Bruce RA, Lindskog BD, Almes MJ, Belanger L, Green B. Treadmill test responses to an early exercise programme after myocardial infarction: A randomized study. Circulation 1982; 65:1420-1428

47.   Aamot IL, Moholdt T, Amundsen BH, Solberg HS, Morkved S, Stoylen A. Onset of exercise training 14 days after uncomplicated myocardial infarction: A randomized controlled trial. Eur J Cardiovasc Prev Rehabil 2010; 17:387-392

48.   Report of the WHO consultation, definition, diagnosis and classification of diabetes mellitus and its complications. Part 1: Diagnosis and classification of diabetes mellitus. World Health Organisation, Department of Non-communicable Disease Surveillance, Geneva 1999.

49.   American Diabetes Association. Diagnosis and classification of diabetes mellitus. Diabetes Care 2008; 31 (Suppl 1): S55-S60

50.   Mezzani A, Hamm LF, Jones AM, et al. Aerobic exercise intensity assessment and prescription in cardiac rehabilitation. J Cardiopulm Rehabil Prev 2012;32:327-350

51.   Mahoney FI, Barthel DN. Functional evolution: The Barthel Index. Md Med J 1965; 14: 61–5

52.   Sainsbury A, Seebass G, Bansal A et al. Reliability of the Barthel index when used with older people. Age Ageing 2005; 34: 228–32

53.   American Thoracic Society (ATS Committee on Proficiency Standards for Clinical Pulmonary Function Laboratories). ATS statement: Guidelines for the six-minute walk test. Am J Respir Crit Care Med 2002;166:111-117

54.   Gibbons RJ, Balady GJ, Bricker JT, et al. ACC/AHA 2002 guideline update for exercise testing: summary article: a report of the American College of Cardiology/American Heart Association Task Force on Practice Guidelines J Am Coll Cardiol 2002;40:1531-1540

55.   Balady GJ, Arena R, Sietsema K, et al. Clinicians guide to cardiopulmonary exercise testing in adults. Circulation 2010;122:191-225

56.   Russo N, Compostella L, Setzu T, et al. Cardiac rehabilitation after transcatheter aortic valve implantation: a single centre experience. Eur Heart J 2011; 32:184

57.   Russo N, Compostella L, Tarantini G, et al. Cardiac rehabilitation after transcatheter versus surgical prosthetic valve implantation for aortic stenosis in the elderly. Eur J Prev Cardiol 2014; 21:1341-48

58.   Bellotto F, Russo N, Compostella L, et al. Cardiac rehabilitation in patients with ventricular assist devices. G Ital Cardiol 2010; 11: 59

59.   Russo N, Compostella L, Setzu T, et al. Intensive, exercise based, cardiac rehabilitation in patients with jarvik 2000 ventricular assist device. Eur J Prev Cardiol 2012; 19: S126

60.   Russo N, Compostella L, Setzu T, et al. Effects of short-term exercise training at anaerobic threshold in patients with axialflow left ventricular assist device. Eur J Prev Cardiol 2013; 20: S30

61.   Compostella L, Russo N, Setzu T, et al. Cardiac autonomic dysfunction in the early phase after left ventricular assist device implant: Implications for surgery and follow-up. Int J Artif Organs 2013; 36: 410-418

62.   Compostella L, Russo N, Setzu T, et al. Exercise Performance of Chronic Heart Failure Patients in the Early Period of Support by an Axial-Flow Left Ventricular Assist Device as Destination Therapy. Artif Organs 2014; 38: 366-373

63.   Russo N, Compostella L, Setzu T, et al. Safety and efficacy of intensive, exercise based, cardiac rehabilitation early after an acute myocardial infarction. Eur J Prev Cardiol 2012; 19: S87

64.   Russo N, Compostella L, Vettore E, et al. Intensive, exercise based, cardiac rehabilitation immediately after an acute myocardial infarction in high risk patients: impact on immediate and long-term prognosis. Eur J Prev Cardiol 2013; 20: S139

65.   Lavie CJ, Milani RV: Effects of cardiac rehabilitation and exercise training programs in patients _75 years of age. Am J Cardiol 1996;78:675-7

66.   Balady GJ, Jette D, Scheer J, et al. Changes in exercise capacity following cardiac rehabilitation in patients stratified according to age and gender. Results of the Massachusetts Association of Cardiovascular and Pulmonary Rehabilitation Multicenter Database. J Cardiopulm Rehabil 1996;16:38-46

67.   Eder B, Hofmann P, Duvillard SP, et al. Early 4-week cardiac rehabilitation exercise training in elderly patients after heart surgery. J Cardiopulm Rehabil Prev 2010;30:85-92

68.   Macchi C, Fattirolli F, Molino Lova R, et al. Early and late rehabilitation and physical training in elderly patients after cardiac surgery. Am J Phys Med Rehabil 2007; 86: 826-834

69. Gotzmann M, Hehen T, Germing A, et al. Short term effects of transcatheter aortic valve implantation on neurohormonal activation, quality of life and 6-minute walk test in severe and symptomatic aortic stenosis. Heart 2010; 96:1102-1106

70. Bagur R, Rodés-Cabau J, Dumont E, et al. Performance-based functional assessment of patients undergoing transcatheter aortic valve implantation. Am Heart J 2011;161:726 –734

71. Passantino A, Lagioia R, Mastropasqua F, et al. Short-term change in distance walked in 6 min is an indicator of outcome in patients with chronic heart failure in clinical practice. J Am Coll Cardiol 2006;48:99-105

72. Russo N, Compostella L, Setzu T, et al. Impact of metabolic syndrome on functional recovery after cardiac rehabilitation. Eur Heart J 2011; 32:711

73. Russo N, Compostella L, Fadini G, et al. Prediabets influences cardiac rehabilitation in coronary artery disease patients. Eur J Prev Cardiol. 2012;19:382-8

74. Scardovia AB, Coletta C, De Maria R, et al. The cardiopulmonary exercise test is safe and reliable in elderly patients with cronic heart failure. J Cardiovasc Med 2007; 8:608-12

75. Lund LH, Mancini D. Peak VO2 in elderly patients with heart failure. Int J Cardiol 2008; 125:166-71

76. Bellotto F, Palmisano P, Russo N, et al. Anemia does not preclude increments in cardiac performance during a short period of intensive, exercise-based cardiac rehabilitation. Eur J Cardiovasc Prev Rehabil 2011;18:150-7

77. Kumpati GS, McCarthy PM, Hoercher KJ. Left Ventricular Assist Device Bridge to Recovery: A Review of the Current Status. Ann Thorac Surg 2001; 71:S103–8

78.   Burkhoff D, Klotz S, Mancini DM. LVAD-induced reverse remodeling: basic and clinical implications for myocardial recovery. J Cardiac Fail 2006; 12:227-239

79.   Jaski BE, Lingle RJ, Reardon LC, Dembitsky WP. Left ventricular assist device as a bridge to patient and myocardial recovery. Prog Cardiovasc Dis 2000; 43:5-18

80.   Mishra V, Fiane AE, Geiran O, et al. Hospital costs fell as numbers of LVADs were increasing: experiences from Oslo University Hospital. J Cadiothorac Surg 2012; 7:76

81.   Laoutaris ID, Dritsas A, Adamopoulos S, et al. Benefits of physical training on exercise capacity, inspiratory muscle function, and quality of life in patients with ventricular assist devices long-term postimplantation. Eur J Cardiovasc Prev Rehabil 2011; 18:33-40

82.   Dimopoulos S, Diakos N, Tseliou E, Tasoulis A, Mpouchla A, Manetos C, Katsaros L, Drakos S, Terrovitis J, Nanas S. Chronotropic incompetence and abnormal heart rate recovery early after left ventricular assist device implantation. Pacing Clin Electrophysiol 2011; 34:1607-1614

83.   Mikus E, Stephanenko A, Krabatsch T, Loforte A, Dandel M, Lehmkuhl HB, Hetzer R, Potapov EV. Reversibility of fixed pulmonary hypertension in left ventricular assist device support recipients. Eur J Cardiothorac Surg 2011; 40:971-977

84.   Cohen-Solal A, Laperche T, Morvan D, Geneves M, Caviezel B, Gourgon R. Prolonged kinetics of recovery of oxygen consumption after maximal graded exercise in patients with chronic heart failure. Analysis with gas exchange measurements and NMR spectroscopy. Circulation 1995; 91:2924-2932

85.   Bellotto F, Compostella L, Agostoni P, Russo N, et al. Peripheral adaptation mechanisms in physical training and cardiac rehabilitation.

The case of a patient supported by a cardiowest total artificial heart. Journal of Cardiac Failure 2011; 17:670-675

86.   Kalra PR, Bolger AP, Francis DP, Genth-Zotz S, Sharma R, Ponikowski PP, Poole-Wilson PA, Coats AJ, Anker SD. Effect of anemia on exercise tolerance in chronic heart failure in men. Am J Cardiol 2003; 91:888–891

87.   Anand IS. Anemia and chronic heart failure implications and treatment options. J Am Coll Cardiol 2008; 52:501–511

88.   Piepoli MF, Guazzi M, Boriani G, et al; Exercise intolerance in chronic heart failure: mechanisms and therapies. Part I. Eur J Cardiovasc Prev Rehabil 2010; 17:637-42

89.   Agostoni P, Salvioni E, Debenedetti C, et al. Relationship of resting hemoglobin concentration to peak oxygen uptake in heart failure patients. Am J Hematol 2010; 85:414-7

90.   Triposkiadis F, Karayannis G, Giamouzis G, Skoularigis J, Louridas G, Butler J. The sympathetic nervous system in heart failure. Physiology, pathophysiology, and clinical implications. J Am Coll Cardiol 2009; 54:1747-62

91.   Olshansky B, Sabbah HN, Hauptman PJ, Colucci WS. Parasympathetic nervous system and heart failure: pathophysiology and potential implications for therapy. Circulation 2008; 118:863-71

92.   Ogletree-Hughes ML, Stull LB, Sweet WE, et al. Mechanical unloading restores beta-adrenergic responsiveness and reverses receptor downregulation in the failing human heart. Circulation 2001; 104:881-6.

93.   Klotz S, Barbone A, Reiken S, et al. Left ventricular assist device support normalizes left and right ventricular beta-adrenergic pathway properties. J Am Coll Cardiol 2005; 45:668-76.

94.   Xydas S, Rosen RS, Ng C, et al. Mechanical unloading leads to echocardiographic, electrocardiographic, neurohormonal, and histologic recovery. J Heart Lung Transplant 2006; 25:7-15.

95.   Kim SY, Montoya A, Zbilut JP, et al. Effect of Heart-Mate left ventricular assist device on cardiac autonomic nervous activity. Ann Thorac Surg 1996; 61:591-3.

96.   Miyagawa S, Sawa Y, Fukushima N, et al. Analysis of sympathetic nerve activity in end-stage cardiomyopathy patients receiving left ventricular support. J Heart Lung Transplant 2001; 20:1181-7.

97.   Soares PPS, Moreno AM, Cravo SLD, Nóbrega ACL. Coronary artery bypass surgery and longitudinal evaluation of the autonomic cardiovascular function. Critical Care 2005; 9:R124-31

98.   Amar D, Fleisher M, Pantuck CB, et al. Persistent alterations of the autonomic nervous system after noncardiac surgery. Anesthesiology 1998; 89:30-42

99.   Vongvanich P, Paul-Labrador MJ, Merz CN. Safety of medically supervised exercise in a cardiac rehabilitation centre. Am J Cardiol 1996;77:1383-1385

100.   Pavy B, Iliou MC, Meurin P, et al. Functional Evaluation and Cardiac Rehabilitation Working Group of the French Society of Cardiology. Safety of exercise training for cardiac patients: Results of the french registry of complications during cardiac rehabilitation. Arch Intern Med 2006;166:2329-2334

101.   Kwan G, Balady G. Cardiac rehabilitation 2012: advancing the field through emerging science. Circulation. 2012;125:369–373.

102.   Williams MA, Haskell WL, Ades PA, et al. Resistance exercise in individuals with and without cardiovascular disease: 2007 update: A scientific statement from the american heart association council on

clinical cardiology and council on nutrition, physical activity, and metabolism. Circulation 2007;116:572-584

103. Gremeaux V, Troisgros O, Benaim S, et al. Determining the minimal clinically important difference for the six-minute walk test and the 200-meter fast-walk test during cardiac rehabilitation programme in coronary artery disease patients after acute coronary syndrome. Arch Phys Med Rehabil 2011;92:611-619

104. Barth J, Critchley J, Bengel J. Efficacy of psychosocial interventions for smoking cessation in patients with coronary heart disease: A systematic review and meta-analysis. Ann Behav Med 2006;32:10-20

105. Perez GH, Nicolau JC, Romano BW, et al. Depression: A predictor of smoking relapse in a 6-month follow-up after hospitalization for acute coronary syndrome. Eur J Cardiovasc Prev Rehabil 2008;15:89-94

106. Kripalani S, Yao X, Haynes RB. Interventions to enhance medication adherence in chronic medical conditions: A systematic review. Arch Intern Med 2007;167:540-550

107. Kim C, Kim DY, Lee DW. The impact of early regular cardiac rehabilitation programme on myocardial function after acute myocardial infarction. Ann Rehabil Med 2011;35:535-540

108. Olivari Z, Steffenino G, Savonitto S, et al. (on behalf of BLITZ 4 Investigators). The management of acute myocardial infarction in the cardiological intensive care units in Italy: the 'BLITZ 4 Qualità' campaign for performance measurement and quality improvement. European Heart Journal: Acute Cardiovascular Care 2012; 1:143-52

109. Coles AH, Fisher KA, Darling C, et al. Recent trends in post-discharge mortality among patients with an initial acute myocardial infarction. Am J Cardiol 2012;110:1073-7

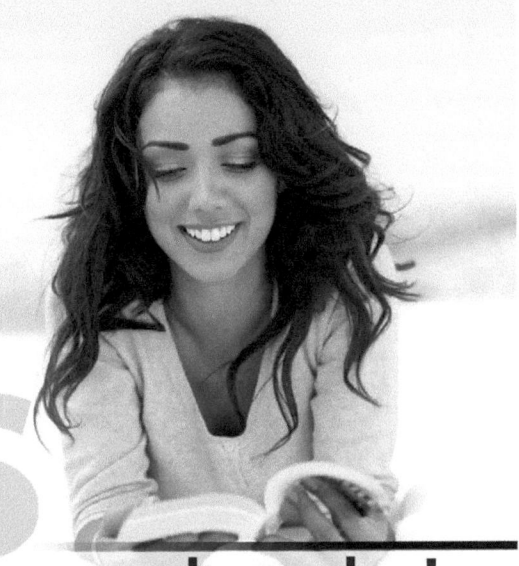 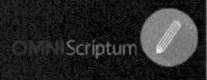

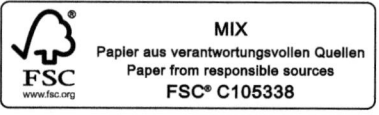

Printed by Books on Demand GmbH, Norderstedt / Germany